Endometriosis

A NATURAL APPROACH

Jo Mears

Ulysses Press Berkeley, CA
1998

Published by: Ulysses Press
P.O. Box 3440
Berkeley, CA 94703-3440

Library of Congress Catalog Card Number: 97-61007

ISBN: 1-56975-088-2

First published as *Coping with Endometriosis* by Sheldon Press

Printed in Canada by Best Book Manufacturers

10 9 8 7 6 5 4 3 2 1

Editor: Mark Woodworth
Cover Design: Leslie Henriques and Sarah Levin
Cover Illustration: "Nude #3" Diana Ong/Super Stock
Editorial and production staff: Lily Chou, Natasha Lay
Typesetter: David Wells
Indexer: Sayre Van Young

Distributed in the United States by Publishers Group West and in Canada by Raincoast Books

Acknowledgments

I would very much like to thank Diane Carlton, Kim Longlands, Dr. B. I. Pirzada and Dr. Michael Brush of the National Endometriosis Society for their help and support, as well as all the women suffering from endometriosis who kindly told me their stories.

Contents

Preface

I am pleased to be able to publish Jo Mears' book *Endometriosis: A Natural Approach*. As a sufferer, I know only too well the anguish that this disease can cause. It not only scars our bodies physically, but it can scar us emotionally as well.

I spent much of my twenties and thirties searching for an answer to why I had abdominal pain. When I had my period it was excruciating; the rest of the month the pain was just there. I endured shots of hydrocortisone in my stomach, pelvic examinations that made me scream in agony, and jeers from both male and female gynecologists. I went from doctor to doctor only to be humiliated and written off as a hypochondriac or "nut case." When I finally was diagnosed with endometriosis, after the scarring was so severe it was palpable to the touch, I actually felt relieved. After all the recriminations, the pain wasn't in my head.

So when I read Jo Mears' book I wanted to be able to share her insights with others so that they could avoid the degradation and delayed diagnosis I had encountered. Her book made me feel that you can cope with the disease no matter how severe it is, and it offered approaches that nurtured and empowered as well as healed.

Her book begins with a clear description of what endometriosis is, and then offers the latest theories about what causes the disease (doctors and scientists are still debating) and how one can go about getting a correct diagnosis. Then it goes a step beyond the average self-help book on the topic. It not only makes accessible detailed information on traditional forms of treatment, such as drugs and therapy, but goes on to offer natural therapies that complement Western medicine. For instance, the book describes how some women who have suffered from endometriosis can break the vicious cycle of pain–depression–more pain by incorporating relaxation techniques into their daily lives. It tells how aromatherapy has increased pain-free days by 59 percent in women studied in Great Britain, how ginger tea can relieve spasms and improve circulation, and how meditation can relax tension, which then relieves pain. One chapter provides coping strategies offering specific methods for easing pain through exercise, flotation therapy, and massage, to name just a few.

Most importantly, this book will likely validate your experience with endometriosis as it did mine. And it comforts by relaying the ordeals and wisdom of other sufferers in a nonjudgmental fashion. The book can be shared with family members (and physicians) so that they, too, can understand what occurs in the course of this affliction. Finally, it supplies lists of support groups and resources for alternative therapies as vehicles to help manage this bewildering disease.

I hope you find this book as helpful as I did.

Leslie Henriques, MPH
Publisher

PART ONE
The Background

CHAPTER ONE

What Is Endometriosis?

Some Basic Facts and Figures

What Does Endometriosis Mean?

If you mention the word endometriosis to most people, they'll look at you with a blank face and say, "Endo *what?*" But on occasion you'll find someone who says, "Oh yes. I've heard of that. My aunt has it. It has to do with painful periods, doesn't it?"

Painful periods are one of the main symptoms of endometriosis, but the name itself is actually derived from the following ancient Greek words:

- *End*, meaning inside
- *Metra*, meaning womb (uterus)
- *Osis*, meaning disease, problem or abnormality

What Is Endometriosis?

As its name suggests, endometriosis is an abnormality connected with the uterus. Endometriosis is a condition that occurs when the tissue that lines the uterus (the endometrium), and that is shed each month during a menstrual period, grows outside the uterus. When anything in the body is found outside its normal site, it is called "ectopic." So you may hear people say that endometriosis is caused by "ectopic endometrium."

How Many Women Are Affected?

It is estimated that 10 percent of women are affected, although some experts believe it could be as many as 20 percent. It is the second most common gynecological condition after fibroid tumors.

Who Is Affected?

Endometriosis most commonly affects women between the ages of 25 to 40. But because it is linked to the monthly cycle, it can occur anytime after your period starts to when it ends (and in some women it even continues after menstruation has stopped). New research suggests that all women may have deposits of endometriosis but that for reasons that are not yet fully understood it only causes a problem in some women.

Why Is It More Common Today?

Endometriosis was first discovered in 1860 by an Austrian physician, von Rokitansky, but it wasn't named until 1924 when Dr. A. J. Sampson described the condition and gave it a name.

That doesn't mean to say that endometriosis didn't exist before then! In fact, many endometriosis sufferers today believe their grandmothers may have suffered with the condition because they remember their having very painful periods (one of the main symptoms).

However, as endometriosis usually regresses during pregnancy, it may have been less common in the past, when most women spent a lot of

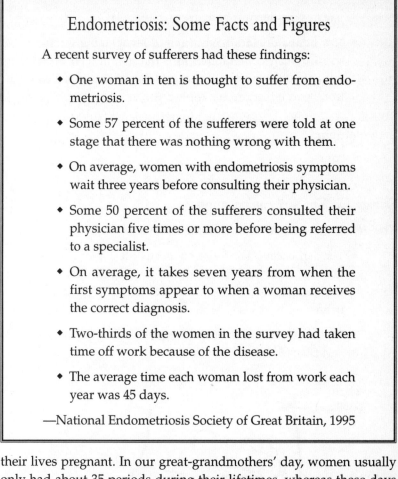

Endometriosis: Some Facts and Figures

A recent survey of sufferers had these findings:

- One woman in ten is thought to suffer from endometriosis.

- Some 57 percent of the sufferers were told at one stage that there was nothing wrong with them.

- On average, women with endometriosis symptoms wait three years before consulting their physician.

- Some 50 percent of the sufferers consulted their physician five times or more before being referred to a specialist.

- On average, it takes seven years from when the first symptoms appear to when a woman receives the correct diagnosis.

- Two-thirds of the women in the survey had taken time off work because of the disease.

- The average time each woman lost from work each year was 45 days.

—National Endometriosis Society of Great Britain, 1995

their lives pregnant. In our great-grandmothers' day, women usually only had about 35 periods during their lifetimes, whereas these days the average woman has about 400 periods. Because endometriosis is associated with menstrual bleeding, it may be that the more periods you have, the more opportunity endometriosis has to develop.

Other reasons for the increase are:

- Doctors are better at diagnosing endometriosis because they are becoming more aware of the condition (although the situation is still far from perfect).

- Doctors have easier means of diagnosing the disease, through a laparoscopy—a telescopic investigation whereby a doctor can actually see the endometriosis patches inside your body (see Chapter 4).

• Nowadays doctors have ways of recognizing microscopic patches of endometriosis that might have been missed in the past and that can cause just as much trouble as larger, more visible areas.

• Women are more assertive today and less afraid of reporting their symptoms, which include painful intercourse.

Where Do You Get Endometriosis?

The most common places for endometriosis to occur are:

• The *peritoneum:* The loose connective tissue of the abdominal cavity, which is a kind of thin skin that protects the organs, allowing them to move freely in the pelvis.

• On the surfaces of the pelvic organs such as the *ovaries* and *fallopian tubes.*

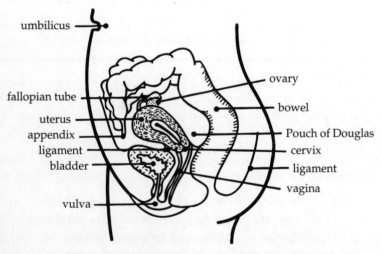

Figure 1: *Endometriosis hot-spots in the pelvis.*

- On the surfaces of the *bowel, bladder* and *intestines.*

- In the *Pouch of Douglas* (a small flap and space behind the uterus, located between the uterus and the rectum). Endometriosis cells often settle here due to the pull of gravity. Doctors can often tell through an internal examination whether there is tenderness there—a sign that endometriosis is probably present.

- Endometriosis has even been known to travel farther afield—to the lungs, nose, ears and even behind the eye—but this is far less common. In fact, it has been found just about everywhere in the body apart from the spleen (see Figure 1 for endometriosis hot-spots).

What Damage Does Endometriosis Do?

Endometriosis hot-spots act like small patches of uterine lining and respond to the hormonal cycles that affect the uterus. This means that these patches bleed during a monthly period. Because the blood has nowhere to go, it collects in the surrounding tissues.

This stray blood sometimes causes local irritation, leading to *inflammation* and *scarring.* In severe cases, it can even produce *solid nodules* or *cysts.* (These include the large "chocolate" cysts sometimes found on the ovaries—called chocolate because of the color caused by the dark blood collecting inside them.)

This damage can also lead to the pelvic organs' becoming stuck together, which doctors refer to as *adhesions.* An adhesion is a web of scar tissue resembling plastic wrap that causes organs to stick together. These adhesions can cause intense pain during menstrual periods and may also affect other pelvic areas such as the bowel, bladder, ovaries and fallopian tubes. (Damage to these areas may affect a woman's fertility as well.)

Some endometriosis hot-spots can also be trapped inside the muscles of the uterine wall (a condition called *adenomyosis*). These spots in the muscle wall can swell and cause more pain.

But to understand more about how endometriosis affects us, we need to understand more about how our bodies work.

How Your Body Works

Let's first of all look at some of the different parts of the body that make up the reproductive organs.

On the Outside

Vulva: The fleshy area around the openings of the vagina and the urethra (the tube leading from the bladder through which you urinate).

Labia: Flaps of skin, like lips, that form the entrance to the vagina.

Clitoris: A small, elongated erectile organ at the front part of the vulva that is very sensitive and that swells during sexual arousal.

On the Inside

Vagina: The passage leading from the opening of the vulva to the cervix of the uterus. This elastic, muscular tube expands and contracts to make room for anything from a tampon to a penis—and even a baby!

Cervix: The neck of the uterus that protrudes into the vagina and that, when touched, feels a bit like the tip of the nose in some women.

Uterus (also known as the *womb*): A hollow, muscular organ located in the pelvis in which the fertilized egg implants and develops. Although thick and muscular, it's normally the size and shape of a pear, but expands during pregnancy. At the top, the uterus branches out into the fallopian tubes on either side. The uterus usually tilts forward toward the bladder, but in women with endometriosis it can tilt backward (called "retroverted"—see more about this in Chapter 2).

Ligaments: These are bands of strong tissue that keep the uterus in place. They stretch across the pelvic cavity from the pelvic walls, the bladder and the rectum. The uterus, the fallopian tubes and the ovaries are all attached to these ligaments, but they should still be able to move easily around and not be firmly stuck in one place (as can often happen with endometriosis).

Fallopian tubes: A pair of slender ducts through which the eggs pass from the ovaries to the uterus. At their ends are fingerlike projections called *fimbriae* that stretch toward the ovaries and catch the eggs when they are released from the ovaries. They're also lined with tiny, hairlike structures called *cilia*, which waft the egg down toward the uterus.

Ovaries: Each about the size of a walnut, these two organs are where the eggs, together with the female sex hormones estrogen and progesterone, are produced. Women are born with eggs already in place, but their numbers drop to about 200,000 to 500,000 by puberty. Every month a number are stimulated to develop by hormones, but only one egg becomes fully developed and is released.

Ovarian follicles: These are the fluid-filled sacs or glands in the ovaries that contain thousands of immature cells that grow into eggs if they are given the correct stimulus.

How Do Your Periods Start?

Your first period is the result of your ovaries' being "switched on" by hormones produced by the pituitary gland (see below).

Where Do Hormones Come From?

The hormones involved in the menstrual cycle come from three different places:

- The *hypothalamus*, part of the brain just above the pituitary gland that controls the body's hormone activity, including stimulation of the pituitary in the menstrual cycle.

- The *pituitary gland*, a pea-sized organ at the base of the skull that produces a hormone that regulates the functioning of the ovaries (among other things).

- The *ovaries*, the place where the eggs are produced.

Facts About Menstrual Periods

Girls start their periods somewhere between 10 and 16, although it can sometimes be earlier or later. The average age is 13.4.

The average age for stopping menstruation is 51, but it can occur earlier or later.

The average number of periods a woman has a year is 13. The menstrual cycle is usually calculated by the medical profession as 28 days long—28 days from the start of one period (called Day 1) until the start of the next one. But in practice, a normal cycle can be anywhere from 21 to 35 days long.

A period can last from one to eight days, although three to five days is more common.

What Do Hormones Do?

A hormone is a chemical that sends messages to different parts of our body telling them to act in a certain way. Our periods are controlled and regulated by several different hormones, which are produced by the parts of the body mentioned above.

What Happens During the Menstrual Cycle?

For our purposes we will assume that the menstrual cycle lasts 28 days. Day 1 is the first day of a period and Day 28 the last period-free day before bleeding starts again.

THE MENSTRUAL PHASE (DAYS 1–5)

1. The hypothalamus produces GnRH (*gonadotrophin*), a releasing hormone that stimulates the pituitary gland.

2. The pituitary in turn is stimulated into producing a hormone called FSH (*follicle-stimulating hormone*).

3. FSH acts on the ovarian follicles, stimulating the eggs into ripening and producing the female hormone called *estrogen*.

THE FOLLICULAR PHASE (DAYS 6–12)

1. Estrogen levels in the blood then rise and are carried in the bloodstream to the uterus where they cause the uterus to start thickening.

2. FSH stops being produced when the uterus is thick enough, and another hormone, LH (*luteinizing hormone*), starts to be released.

3. LH then triggers the ovulatory phase.

THE OVULATORY PHASE (DAYS 13–15)

1. LH causes one of the maturing follicles to burst and release an egg. At this time some women feel pain, which doctors call *Mittelschmerz*, literally meaning "pain in the middle."

2. By this time, the open ends of the fallopian tubes have moved closer to the ovaries, making them ready to catch the released egg.

3. The cilia hairs that line the fallopian tubes waft the egg down one of the tubes and into the uterus. (At this time the vaginal mucus thins, enabling sperm to swim more easily.)

THE LUTEAL PHASE (DAYS 16–23)

By the time the egg has wafted down the tube, this phase has already begun.

1. After the collapse of the ovarian follicle, cells proliferate and form a yellow cyst called the *corpus luteum* (meaning "yellow body"). The corpus luteum then begins its own hormone production, starting to manufacture another female hormone called *progesterone*.

2. Progesterone stops any more ovarian follicles from ripening, and helps to further develop the uterus, making it soft and spongy and secreting nourishment for when the egg arrives.

3. The uterus continues to thicken as the egg spends another seven to eight days traveling down to the uterus. To become fertilized, the egg must meet live sperm in the first 12 to 24 hours after the egg is released and before it begins to decay. (Vaginal mucus is thick at this time to prevent additional sperm from entering.)

4. If the egg is fertilized by a sperm, it in turn secretes another hormone into the bloodstream called HCG (*human chorionic gonadotrophin*), which stimulates the corpus luteum to go on making progesterone, which in turn makes the uterus develop even further. Progesterone production is eventually taken over by the placenta and continues throughout pregnancy to stop the uterine lining from being shed.

5. However, if the egg is not fertilized, no HCG is produced, the corpus luteum breaks down after seven days, and progesterone production stops.

THE PREMENSTRUAL PHASE (DAYS 24–28)

1. Estrogen and progesterone levels fall sharply.

2. During the following seven days, in response to the drop in progesterone levels, the muscles in the uterine walls spasm and cut off the blood supply to the uterus. This causes the lining to break down and to be expelled as a menstrual period. Usually two-thirds of the uterine lining is shed, while the remaining one-third—a basic, deep layer—remains.

3. At the end of a menstrual period, progesterone and estrogen levels are at their lowest in the blood, which

triggers the production of GnRH again, and then FSH and LH. And so the whole cycle starts again!

What Goes Wrong in Women with Endometriosis?

When the uterus responds to hormonal changes it sheds its endometrial lining through the vagina. However, endometrial tissue residing outside the uterus has no way of escaping the body, which results in internal bleeding that may cause inflammation and scarring of the surrounding areas. Other organs, such as the bladder or bowel in the pelvis, are often involved.

What Is Menstrual Blood?

The top two-thirds of the uterine lining (the endometrium) is shed during a period; it includes red blood cells, mucus, hormones, hormonelike structures called *prostaglandins,* and tissue debris. Our main interest is in the live endometrial cells from the uterine lining that are thought to attach themselves to other areas in the pelvis, and that then begin to grow.

What Is Endometrial Tissue?

Endometrial tissue is uterine lining that can cause a problem when it is found outside the uterus. It appears in several different forms: as we discussed earlier, it can form as microscopic patches, cysts or nodules. Whatever form the endometriosis takes, the tissue it produces is made up of cells similar to the lining of the uterus. They are often referred to by different names, but basically they are all the same thing: endometrial tissue, patches, deposits, spots or implants; or endometriotic blisters, lesions, vesicles or cells.

Is Endometriosis Life Threatening?

One of the biggest worries when women are first diagnosed with endometriosis is whether the condition is life threatening in any way. Women with endometriosis can in theory die from related complications—such as septicemia resulting from an obstructed bowel—but it isn't likely, and fortunately there are no known cases of a woman dying directly as a result of endometriosis. The major problem with endometriosis is that it's a chronic condition, involving very slow changes. And it can be very painful and debilitating. This book will help you understand it and learn to cope with it, using natural approaches.

CHAPTER TWO

What Causes Endometriosis?

No one knows for sure what causes endometriosis. However, tests on endometrial cells found outside the uterus have shown that endometrial cells are similar to those in the uterine lining. But just how they got there isn't really clear.

Some researchers believe that women with endometriosis are born with endometrial deposits in places other than the uterus, while others presume these cells somehow shifted there from the uterus in later life.

There are many more theories in addition to these. However, no single theory has been proven, and it is highly likely that endometriosis could be the result of a combination of any number of them. Here are some of the theories in a bit more detail.

Retrograde Menstruation

The most prevalent and oldest theory is that endometriosis is caused by retrograde menstruation (when some of the menstrual blood flows backward in the wrong direction). It is thought that muscle spasms during a menstrual period sometimes force the menstrual blood backward up through the fallopian tubes and out into the pelvic cavity.

To understand this theory you need to remember the nature of your reproductive organs. As you might recall from the diagram in Chapter 1, the vagina leads up to the cervix, which then leads into the uterus. The top of the uterus then branches out into the fallopian tubes on either side, which are directed toward the ovaries. In many diagrams, the fallopian tubes seem to join up with the ovary, but in fact there is a gap between them. When an egg is released from the ovaries each month, it avoids this gap because it is protected by the small fingerlike projections (fimbriae) that direct the egg into the fallopian tubes.

But when menstrual blood is forced back up the fallopian tubes by muscle spasms during a period, it *does* slip down this gap into the pelvic cavity. This theory is backed up by research that shows that some of this stray menstrual blood contains active cells from the uterine lining that are then thought to implant themselves elsewhere in the pelvic cavity.

A brief summary of some of the experiments that support this theory includes the following:

- Many cases of endometriosis are found in the lower part of the pelvis, which is the obvious place for the stray blood to collect. Also, a lot of endometrial deposits are found near the ends of the fallopian tubes, which are the closest sites to the gap.

- In experiments, endometrial cells have been planted in the peritoneal cavity (the membrane of the abdominal cavity) and have taken root there and grown.

- Live endometrial cells have been found in menstrual blood as well as in the fallopian tubes and peritoneal fluid.

- The female hormones estrogen and progesterone have been found to be important for the long-term survival of endometrial implants.

- Women with a tight or closed-off cervical canal appear to be more likely to get endometriosis. In other words, the buildup of pressure in the uterus could cause menstrual blood to flow backward.

- Most women having periods have been found to have a certain amount of retrograde menstruation. In one study of women having "keyhole surgery" (laparoscopy) during their period, 90 percent of those with normal fallopian tubes were found to have quite a lot of blood in their peritoneal cavity.

The question is, why do stray endometrial cells in menstrual blood take root in some women and not in others? If you read on, the autoimmune system theory may offer a potential explanation for this.

Autoimmune Theory

This is another common theory. Many scientists believe that the immune system plays a key role in endometriosis. It's thought that a healthy immune system usually prevents normal body cells from implanting themselves in unusual sites. Stray endometrial cells found in the pelvic cavity would normally be eaten up or destroyed by the body's own natural defenses, and therefore wouldn't be able to implant themselves. However, for some reason this system either doesn't work or overreacts in endometriosis sufferers. Researchers also think this alteration in the immune system might be passed on from generation to generation.

Other Theories

Bloodstream Theory

Some researchers believe that live endometrial cells somehow pass into the bloodstream during a menstrual period and travel around the body. They say this accounts for the fact that endometriosis is sometimes found in unusual sites that have a rich blood supply, such as the lungs or body muscles.

Lymphatic Theory

This theory suggests that live endometrial cells somehow pass into the lymphatic system during a period. The lymphatic system is a complete system of vessels (like blood vessels) that carry nutrients to and from tissues and that also help to keep the immune system working. Some scientists say that this explains why endometriosis is sometimes found in lymphatic areas, such as around the navel, which is rich in lymphatic vessels draining the pelvic area.

Waste Ova Theory

This theory suggests that some of the eggs that are released every month slip down in the gap between the fallopian tubes and ovaries, and that some of the cells attached to the egg develop into endometriosis sites, under certain hormonal conditions.

Embryonic Cell Rests Theory

This theory posits that some female embryos develop duplicate *Mullerian ducts* (the structures in an embryo that eventually develop into adult reproductive organs). These Mullerian cells, which are known as "rests," then develop into patches of functioning endometrium in later life.

Coelomic Metaplasia Theory

Metaplasia means the changing of one type of cell into another. This theory suggests that patches of endometrial cells are formed before birth in places other than the uterus, and that they lie dormant in some women but are somehow activated in endometriosis sufferers. Alternatively, normal cells are thought to change suddenly into endometrial cells, triggered perhaps by contact with stray endometrial cells.

Surgical Causes

Certain surgeries, such as cesarean sections, D & Cs, hysterectomies or treatment for fibroids, have been linked to triggering endometrio-

Possible Thyroid Link

One researcher, Dr. Michael Brush, believes that some women with endometriosis may be suffering from a thyroid dysfunction. In a survey of the thyroid function and endocrine levels (hormones secreted from glands like the pituitary) of 120 women with endometriosis, he found that, although their routine thyroid tests were normal, the incidence of thyroid autoantibodies was 20 percent higher than the reported percentage incidence rate in other women. In some cases, the levels of thyroid autoantibodies were consistent with a definite thyroid autoimmune disease. Some of these cases were treated with low-dose thyroxine and the women's health improved considerably.

sis because they stir up the bottom lining of the uterus, which could cause it to implant elsewhere.

Dioxins

One new school of thought has looked into the possibility that manufactured chemicals called dioxins may be a cause of endometriosis. Researchers believe that dioxins may behave like hormones, causing estrogen levels to rise. Dioxins are byproducts of manufacturing processes involving chlorine, which include plastics, PVCs, solvents, pesticides, wood preservatives, disinfectants and pharmaceutical drugs. They are produced when the waste containing these chlorines is burned. The dioxins then go into the air and fall onto the grass and plants, where they are then eaten by animals such as cows. Animal fats, such as meat and dairy products, are thought to be the major source of dioxins in humans.

Research suggests that dioxins attack the immune system, causing problems such as low sperm counts in men and a high incidence of endometriosis in women.

Researchers at the Women's Environmental Health Network estimate that dioxins could affect between 1 and 8 percent of unborn babies, and are looking to see how dioxins may affect their fertility in later life. It is also thought that dioxins could lead to change in thyroid function and the immune system.

Heredity: Does Endometriosis Run in Families?

Endometriosis *does* seem to be hereditary. If a close relative (such as a mother, sister or aunt) suffers from endometriosis, you are 7 to 10 percent more likely to acquire it yourself. However, scientists are not yet certain whether this is due to an inherited gene or environmental factors that are "inherited" from our relatives—such as a tendency to smoke or eat certain types of diets. It's also been discovered that women with very close relatives suffering from endometriosis are more likely to get it severely, and that it seems to be passed on through the mother's family.

Other Possible Causes

Delayed Motherhood

Pregnancy is known to protect against endometriosis, because during pregnancy you don't have periods, thus facing less of a chance of retrograde menstruation. It is also thought that the high levels of estrogen and progesterone in the body during pregnancy may somehow protect against endometriosis.

However, if you delay motherhood it doesn't mean that you will definitely suffer from endometriosis. On the other hand, delayed motherhood due to infertility can sometimes be the result of endometriosis, since some women with endometriosis take longer to get pregnant or may not be able to become pregnant (see Chapter 5).

A "Career Woman's" Disease

Doctors often used to refer to endometriosis as the "career woman's" disease, because working women who often delayed motherhood were more frequently reported to be suffering from endometriosis. However, this is now thought to be incorrect, as the early studies didn't take into account such things as attitudes toward menstrual pain or willingness to question a diagnosis. In other words, career women might be more assertive in their complaints. That doesn't mean, however, that noncareer women aren't suffering as well. Indeed, endometriosis has now been found to affect all sectors of society, including teenagers, ethnic minority groups and even postmenopausal women.

> Jacqueline, 34, who was diagnosed as having endometriosis and fibroids, says: "I think there was a delay in my diagnosis because I'm black and I kept getting sent off to the sexually transmitted diseases clinic—even though I'd only had two boyfriends. When I was eventually diagnosed after undergoing a laparoscopy, the doctor looked at me quizzically and said, 'That's strange. You seem too young to get endometriosis.' Having read more about it since, I realize it can affect just about any woman of any age!"

The Position of the Uterus

In most women, the uterus tilts slightly forward and the cervix points slightly backward. But in some women the uterus may be tilted farther forward (anteverted), or be tilted backward (retroverted) with the cervix pointing forward.

Some studies suggest that women with a uterus that tilts backward may be twice as likely to get endometriosis; other experts dispute this. One theory may be that this position makes it easier for cells in retrograde menstruation to settle in the pelvis.

Endometriosis can, in fact, cause problems in women with any type of uterus. However, women who have a retroverted or anteverted uterus may have the added problem of the uterus being fixed in a rigid position because of surrounding adhesions (see Chapter 1 for an explanation of adhesions).

The Pill and the IUD

Some women feel they have made themselves vulnerable to endometriosis because they have been taking birth-control pills, which affects hormones—and we know that hormones play a significant role in endometriosis.

Early versions of the Pill contained relatively large amounts of estrogen, which could have made women more susceptible to endometriosis by increasing the amount of endometrium-stimulating estrogen in the body. But current prescriptions of the Pill, containing higher levels of progesterone, are thought to actually protect against endometriosis. This is because progesterone is the hormone responsible for breaking down the uterus, and that generally also has the effect of softening and breaking down endometrial deposits as well.

There are similar worries about intrauterine devices that, to a certain extent, work as a contraceptive by irritating the uterine lining. But so far, IUDs have not been found to increase the risk of endometriosis.

Tampons

Some women fear that tampons may cause retrograde menstruation by blocking the exit of menstrual blood from the uterus. Again, there is no evidence of this, although teenage girls with obstructions (such as a narrow cervix) have been found to be much more likely to develop endometriosis. If you are worried, you could use sanitary napkins more often, or perhaps just during the night.

> Maria, 32, who suffers from endometriosis in the bladder area, says: "I find that tampons seem to make my menstrual pain worse, and sometimes are even impossible to insert. I'm much happier using sanitary napkins. Sometimes I only use tampons at the end of my period."

Stress

Obviously, anyone suffering pain a great of the time will feel stress—and stress is now known to depress the immune system, slowing down the action of the white blood cells that help to destroy invading organisms. As of yet, the role of stress and the autoimmune dysfunction in endometriosis isn't fully understood, although it is an area of continuing research.

CHAPTER THREE

Do I Have Endometriosis?

What Are the Symptoms?

Pain is the most common symptom of endometriosis and the reason most sufferers go to their doctors. However, the extent of the pain doesn't seem to be dependent on how much endometriosis you have, but rather on where it is. For instance, a small number of cysts in an area that is disturbed during intercourse may be much more painful than a larger number elsewhere. Most sufferers also report that their pain seems to get worse during their period, although many other sufferers also report experiencing constant pain. Generally, however, if the pain comes and goes during your menstrual cycle, it's highly suggestive of endometriosis.

There are five classic symptoms of endometriosis.

- Painful periods (known as *dysmenorrhea*)
- Painful intercourse (*dyspareunia*)

- ◆ Pelvic pain, including painful bowel movements and constipation
- ◆ Infertility
- ◆ Painful urination

Some of the other commonly reported symptoms are:

- ◆ Painful ovulation (known as *Mittelschmerz*)
- ◆ Heavy periods, including loss of blood clots and stale brown blood
- ◆ Abnormal bleeding
- ◆ Depression
- ◆ Premenstrual syndrome
- ◆ Back pain

Painful Menstrual Periods

Many women complain of painful cramps, which often reach their peak two days after their periods have started. But how do you know whether your periods are more painful than anyone else's? This is particularly difficult to tell, since most of us were brought up to think that it's normal for periods to be painful.

Are Your Periods Painful?

The following questions may help you to decide whether your menstrual pain is severe. The more often you answer "Yes," the more likely you are to suffer from menstrual pain caused by endometriosis.

1. Do you take days off work each month because of menstrual cramps?

2. Do you wake up at night because of menstrual cramps?

3. Is your pain so bad that it can't be relieved by over-the-counter painkillers?

    4. Are your menstrual pains getting worse each year?

    5. Does your pain last longer with each period?

This is how some women suffering from endometriosis describe their pain.

> Jennifer, a 40-year-old women's-shelter worker, who was diagnosed with endometriosis and fibroids, says: "The first time I went to my doctor complaining about my menstrual pains, I felt as though my insides were dropping out. I explained that I was often off work for three weeks at a time, and would be crippled by the pain and running a high temperature. During my period, often all I could do was just lie in the bathtub crying."

> Linda, a 28-year-old kitchen designer who discovered she had extensive endometriosis that included her bowel, recalls: "I always have a gripping pain shooting right through my stomach and back, and feel very sick and dizzy. Every month I have to take time off work because of it."

> Lynne, a 38-year-old architectural planner, diagnosed with endometriosis and an ovarian cyst, says, "The pain during my period was so bad that I couldn't go out. And the painkillers the doctor kept prescribing were absolutely useless."

Painful Sex

Painful intercourse is often a leading indicator of endometriosis, because intercourse can disturb endometrial patches or scar tissue in the pelvic area. But understandably, many women are reluctant to mention this symptom to their doctors, which often delays a diagnosis (see Chapter 4).

Do You Have Painful Sex?

You should seek help if you experience any of the following:

    1. You are avoiding intercourse because it hurts during or after sex.

2. You feel a deep pain in your vagina during intercourse.

3. Sex is more painful at certain times of the month or in
   specific positions.

Jennifer says: "My husband and I hadn't had sex for a year and
a half before I finally went to see a gynecologist. If we tried to
have sex, not only would it hurt at that immediate time, but the
pain would go on for days afterward."

Leora, a 29-year-old daycare worker, says: "Sex in certain positions was excruciatingly painful. For me, one night of active sex
meant two weeks of pain afterward."

Jackie, a 33-year-old science administrator who suffers from
severe endometriosis, says: "Sex for me is like making love to
a bayonet. I get pain during and after intercourse, and even
pain with the big 'O'—if I ever get that far! Sometimes I also
bleed afterward. I couldn't understand why it was so painful
until, after a laser laparoscopy, a deeply embedded nodule was
found at the top of the vagina in the wall of tissue between the
vagina and the rectum. I was extremely annoyed because my
gynecologist had previously said to me, 'Some women will
experience painful intercourse, and the reasons aren't always
physical'—which had meant I'd gone on suffering pain for nine
months before the *real* reason was discovered."

Pelvic Pain

Pelvic pain is basically pain located in the pelvic area of the lower abdomen. The pelvis is formed by the hip bones, sacrum and coccyx, and
protects organs such as the bowel, bladder and ovaries. Pain in this
area might occur midcycle when you ovulate and your eggs are released (also known as Mittelschmerz).

Vanessa, a 24-year-old cosmetician, suffered midcycle pain: "I
found that the pain when I was ovulating was the worst," she
says. "It was an excruciating pain all down the right side of my
abdomen. Once, it got so bad that I collapsed and had to be

> rushed to the emergency room. It was the sort of pain that nothing could blot out."

Pelvic pain can also occur before, during and after your period. Some women even complain of experiencing a dull pain in the pelvic area all the time.

> Paula, a 36-year-old mother of two and a part-time healthcare assistant, diagnosed with endometriosis on the ovary and uterine ligaments, says: "In my early twenties I found I was getting pain all the time, which meant I had to take a lot of time off work. If I hadn't been working for such a sympathetic employer I'm sure I would have been fired."

> Megan, a 29-year-old graduate student who has been treated for fibroids and severe endometriosis, comments: "I've had very painful periods ever since I was ten. The pain was excruciating, and by the time I was in my twenties I was experiencing pain for two weeks every month. It was a sort of constant nag, and my abdomen always felt sore. I also felt a sharp pain whenever I sat down, and if I walked it would get worse."

But sometimes this sort of pain can be caused by other conditions that may have to be ruled out first (see the end of this chapter).

Do You Have Pelvic Pain?

The following questions might help. Again, the more times you answer "Yes," the more likely you are to suffer from pelvic pain caused by endometriosis.

1. Do certain movements or positions—such as walking, running, sitting or lying down—cause you pelvic pain?

2. Do you have low back pain before, during or after your period?

3. Does a bowel movement or urination become painful during your period?

Kim, 36, married with one daughter and diagnosed with moderate endometriosis behind the uterus, says: "Ever since I was a teenager I've had terrible periods that have involved constipation and diarrhea. I'd often get constipation for up to ten days before my period started, and would spend hours on the toilet with my mom having to pass me magazines to read while I was sitting there! Once my period started, I'd get diarrhea. My doctor just put it down to me being a neurotic teenager!"

Linda says, "I'd usually get diarrhea leading up to my period and then constipation for three to four days afterward. I also had horrible cystitis-like symptoms during my period, and the pain was almost unbearable when I went to the bathroom. My doctor kept diagnosing a fiber problem. But once, when he wasn't there, someone else sent me for a scan—and later a laparoscopy—that revealed a cyst on my ovary and endometriosis on most of my pelvic organs and bladder, with possible bowel complications that are still being investigated."

Judith, a 53-year-old farmer, says, "I'd never had any problems with periods when suddenly one night I had to get up and go to the bathroom at least three times. I got something from the pharmacist for cystitis, but it didn't help at all. It just got worse and worse. My family doctor eventually diagnosed a urinary infection and put me on an antibiotic. I was then sent to see a urologist and underwent a cystoscopy (a type of bladder examination) and kidney X-rays. When these revealed nothing, I was finally sent to a gynecologist. He suggested endometriosis and put me on danazol; eventually I had a laparoscopy, which revealed endometrial scarring around the bladder area."

Infertility

Between 25 and 50 percent of women investigated for infertility are found to be suffering from endometriosis. However, it's still not clear whether endometriosis causes infertility, whether it's just somehow associated with it or whether it is simply a coincidental finding. The following questions might help you to decide whether your infertility could be associated with endometriosis.

Could You Be Suffering from Infertility?

1. Have you been trying unsuccessfully to get pregnant for more than a year?

2. Have you been having sex only during your fertile periods but still haven't become pregnant?

3. Have you experienced more than one miscarriage?

Helen, a 35-year-old accountant, says, "Since I'd started my periods, they were so painful that I'd often pass out. But it was only when I read an article about painful periods that I wondered whether endometriosis might be the cause. The slight suspicion that I might have endometriosis deepened in my early thirties when I tried for two years to get pregnant without success. I was then advised to have a laparoscopy, and mild endometriosis was diagnosed. But they also said I had a kink in one of my fallopian tubes and that one of my ovaries was quite far from the fallopian tube. I went on drug treatment followed by in vitro fertilization, but eventually became pregnant naturally."

For more information on infertility see Chapter 5.

Other Symptoms

Heavy Periods

Officially, a heavy period is said to occur when over 80 milliliters of blood is lost, but we are hardly likely to get out a measuring cup to see if we fall into this category. However, the following are indicators of a heavy period:

- ◆ Frequent flooding: when your tampon or sanitary napkin is unable to hold the flow and needs to be changed constantly (such as, every two hours).

- ◆ Your menstrual flow includes blood clots: usually blood clots are broken down by a specific enzyme, but when there's a lot of blood it can't keep up and clots appear.

- You are suffering from anemia: this can be due to heavy blood loss.

Kim recalls, "During my period blood would come out as I sat on the toilet as though I were passing urine. I had to change my sanitary napkin every hour, and I would always have to change my sheets because I leaked in bed at night."

Abnormal Bleeding

The following are types of abnormal bleeding that can occur as a result of endometriosis:

- Irregular periods
- Having your periods more often, that is, your cycle gets progressively shorter
- Spotting before your period, or bleeding midcycle
- Dark discharge following your period

Megan says: "In my twenties my cycle seemed to get shorter and shorter, going down from every 29 days to every 23. And most of the time I felt nauseous and in pain."

Whereas Fiona, a 28-year-old office manager, says: "After I came off the Pill in my early twenties, I had horrendous periods that lasted for eight to ten days. They were so bad I could not eat a thing, and I lost a lot of weight."

Depression

Quite high levels of depression are reported by endometriosis sufferers, often because pain can be very hard to cope with. It can make you feel tense and irritable and lead to feeling rundown, depressed and lacking in self-esteem. This, in turn, can lower your pain threshold. Worries about infertility can also add to this. The confusion and lack of understanding about endometriosis may also make you feel that you have no control over the illness. Chapters 6 and 7 deal with some of the ways in which you can break this vicious circle. But in the meantime it may just help to realize that it's a normal reaction, and not to blame yourself for feeling the way you do.

PMS

Endometriosis is thought to be one of the triggers of premenstrual syndrome (PMS)—the name now given to the troublesome symptoms we often feel just before a period. There are more than 150 symptoms now listed for PMS, but some of the most common ones are mood changes, bloating, weight gain, depression and food cravings.

> Irene, a 40-year-old market research assistant, says: "At least ten days before my period I'd get terrible mood swings and tiredness. I felt I couldn't cope, and if I just knocked a cup of coffee over I'd feel like jumping out of the window. I became fanatical about cleaning, and would snap at everyone and pick on my daughter. Also I slept very badly, and had quite a sore chest—bad enough for me not to be able to put my seatbelt on. As soon as my period started, these feelings would lift. When I began to get awful pain down my right side and PMS symptoms at other times of the month, I decided to have a hysterectomy. During the operation my ovaries were found to be riddled with endometriosis."

Back Pain

In one study, constant lower back pain is reported by 42 percent of endometriosis sufferers, while 37 percent only experience it during their periods. In some cases the pain could be due to endometrial deposits around the intestines (that is, the stomach and bowel areas).

> Leora says, "Six months after having laser treatment for an abnormal cervical smear, I began to experience low back pain continually, which became worse on getting out of bed in the morning. I didn't think this pain was cyclical because I had it all the time, and it began to drive me crazy."

Conditions That Are Confused with Endometriosis

One problem with diagnosing endometriosis is that it can easily be confused with other conditions, such as those described below.

Pelvic inflammatory disease (PID): As its name suggests, this is an inflammation of the pelvis usually involving the uterus, fallopian tubes and ovaries. Because it can cause painful sex, nagging pain, and heavy periods, it's often considered the first explanation for these symptoms, especially if you have a history of PID.

Fibroids: These are benign tumors of fibrous or muscular tissue that develop in the wall of the uterus and can cause heavy bleeding and symptoms similar to PID.

Kidney stones: These are calcified deposits in the kidneys that can cause intermittent, sharp pain or a constant dull ache.

Cystitis: This and other urinary tract infections are often confused with endometriosis. Cystitis is basically an infection caused by inflammation of the bladder—making you want to urinate frequently (and painfully).

Ectopic pregnancy: This is where the fetus develops outside the uterus, often in fallopian tubes that are blocked or inflamed. It frequently results in a sudden pain in the stomach area, radiating up to the collar bone.

Crohn's Disease: A chronic condition in which segments of the alimentary tract become inflamed, scarred, thickened and ulcerated.

Irritable bowel syndrome (IBS): This disease causes recurrent abdominal pain along with constipation or diarrhea.

Salpingitis: This is an inflammation of one or both of the fallopian tubes, usually causing a sharp pain in the lower abdomen.

Take Note!

Because the symptoms of endometriosis can (paradoxically) be caused by some of the above conditions, you should seek a doctor's help immediately if you experience any of them. However, once these other conditions have been ruled out, endometriosis should be suspected —especially if your symptoms are cyclical and only seem to occur leading up to or during your menstrual period.

"I WAS MISDIAGNOSED FOR 18 YEARS"

Jennifer says, "It took me 18 years to get a proper diagnosis. I got my first symptoms at 22—symptoms such as a dull ache behind the navel, painful periods and painful sex. The doctor was very unsympathetic; at first he suggested it could be a sexually transmitted disease. Over the years, he diagnosed salpingitis, cystitis, a kidney infection and irritable bowel syndrome. In the end it was a female friend who listened to my symptoms and suggested endometriosis, and I demanded to see a consultant—who discovered I had endometriosis and two fibroids!"

Leora recalls, "The first time I went to the doctor complaining of low back pain and pain after sex, she said it was an infection and put me on a week-long course of antibiotics. When the antibiotics didn't help, she kept on prescribing different courses of antibiotics. Then PID was diagnosed (in spite of negative vaginal swabs!) and a urinary infection (in spite of a urine sample being clear of infection). Then it was irritable bowel syndrome and a suspected ovarian cyst. It was only when I read an article about endometriosis that alarm bells started to ring and I demanded that my doctor send me for a laparoscopy. Mild endometriosis was finally diagnosed. I was so relieved that they had found something and my pain was now being taken seriously. I've since found out that I was actually lucky, because the average delay in diagnosis is about seven years."

Other Terms To Know

You may hear the following terms being used in connection with endometriosis:

Endometrioma: A cyst containing endometrial tissue.

Adenomyosis: A condition characterized by ingrowth of the endometrium into the wall of the uterus.

Ovarian cyst: A fluid-filled sac that develops on the ovary. If cysts become large and twist on their stalks, they can cause severe abdominal pain and vomiting.

Endometrial polyps: Growths in the uterine lining that form on a stalk and can cause pain as they twist.

Endometritis: When the lining of the uterus becomes somehow inflamed, for example by using an IUD.

CHAPTER FOUR

Getting a Diagnosis

Why Is It Important?

It is important to diagnose endometriosis because its treatment is different from that for other gynecological or bowel problems. It is also thought that inflammation and scar tissue build up each month, which can lead to further complications, and in some cases infertility.

Having said that, other studies have shown that endometriosis doesn't always get worse. In fact, some research has shown that endometriosis can resolve itself spontaneously in 25 percent of the cases—and can go from an active to a more passive form in 50 percent of the cases. The problem is that its difficult to tell which women will get better and which will get worse.

Because endometriosis *does* seem to cure itself in some women, there is now an argument for not having treatment, especially if the endometriosis is mild. Whether or not to undergo treatment is a choice that an individual woman has to make after getting proper information about her condition. Some women decide they'll try anything to get rid of the pain, whereas others might want to start with the least drastic treatments and work their way from there.

Why Are There Delays in Diagnosis?

There is an average delay of seven years from the onset of symptoms to getting a correct diagnosis. A number of reasons are given for this, one of the main ones being that women *expect* to get painful periods (one of the most common symptoms) so they aren't aware that anything is wrong. Also, women are often reluctant to seek help, because they are embarrassed by the symptoms, especially if these include painful sex.

What's more, doctors are not always aware of endometriosis and often confuse it with other conditions that have similar symptoms (see Chapter 3). It doesn't help that there isn't one specific symptom that relates solely to endometriosis. It can take a long time to rule out the other conditions first. Also, there are no specific tests to diagnose endometriosis—other than visually, by means of a laparoscope.

> Paula says, "I only found out I had endometriosis after one of my clients (I run a cleaning company) needed a house cleaner because her endometriosis was making it difficult for her to do the cleaning herself. I went along and by the end of the conversation I realized that I probably had endometriosis, too. Everything just sounded so *familiar*."

> Jennifer comments, "It was my beautician who told me I had endometriosis. I was complaining to her that I felt tired all the time, had painful periods and sex that hurt, when she suddenly cried, 'You've got endo!' She then persuaded me to go back to my doctor and ask to see a gynecologist. It was a good thing she did that, because endometriosis and fibroids were diagnosed and I eventually underwent a hysterectomy because of the pain."

Dealing with Doctors

Getting a Referral

If you're a member of an HMO (health maintenance organization), you may have to be referred by your general practitioner to a gynecologist. When you visit your physician, whether your family doctor or the doctor who sees you at your HMO, it's important that you are very clear about *all* your symptoms so that he or she can get a clear picture of what is wrong. It is a good idea to make a list of your symptoms *before* visiting the doctor. (It may help to read Chapter 3 to see if you recognize any of them.) If you feel very embarrassed, you could even give the list to your doctor to read. If the doctor explains things in a complicated manner, don't be scared to ask to have what he or she said repeated in simpler terms.

Many sufferers complain that their doctors didn't take their symptoms seriously at first. If this happens to you, don't be afraid to go back—often doctors take a "wait and see" attitude whereby they expect people to return if their problem is still troubling them. Other sufferers have complained that their doctors thought their conditions were psychosomatic (all in the mind). Some women may truly be suffering from other problems, like depression, but that doesn't mean they aren't also suffering from endometriosis! Besides, as we already know, endometriosis can be very exhausting, leading to tiredness and depression.

Changing Your Doctor

If you really feel your doctor isn't helping, ask to change doctors.

> Diane, 55, a home-health nurse who eventually underwent a hysterectomy for endometriosis, says: "My first GP wasn't at all sympathetic, and when I eventually got hold of my medical chart I was horrified to see he'd written in a letter 'Munchausen's Syndrome' with a question mark (a psychiatric condition where you purposely make yourself appear ill to attract attention). I couldn't believe he would say that, when I'd already

been diagnosed as suffering from endometriosis and had had to have several operations.

"During the discussion, I asked him why he'd written Munchausen's down. His only explanation was that he didn't really understand endometriosis. Although I did change doctors, it makes me angry even now to think that it's still written down in my medical chart."

How to Get the Best from Your Doctor

1. Prepare for the consultation before you go. Think clearly about your symptoms and how they affect your life.

2. Make a list of your symptoms. You can actually take the list with you and read them out if you want.

3. Rehearse what you want to say, either with someone else or just in your own mind.

4. Take someone with you to the consultation for support. Everyone has a right to do this.

5. If you think you'll need longer than usual with your doctor, ask the receptionist if you can arrange for a longer appointment.

6. Take with you the names and regimen of any drugs or medicines you have been taking.

7. If the doctor suggests a physical examination, ask him or her what sort of information this might give. Also remember that you can ask for the examination to stop at any time if you're not happy or feel uncomfortable.

8. If there's anything you don't understand, ask your doctor to explain—as many times as is necessary!

9. If you are prescribed any drugs, ask if there are any side effects you should look out for.

10. If students are to be present during your consultation, the doctor should ask your permission first. You have the right to refuse.

11. If you want to see your medical chart, your doctor can arrange this for you.

Learning to Be Assertive

One of the problems we all have is not being assertive enough with our medical practitioners. When you are feeling tired and rundown, or possibly depressed, it is much harder to stick up for yourself. If you are having problems with asserting yourself and asking for what you want, you could try taking an assertiveness course as an evening class, or speaking to a counselor.

Having said that, remember that your doctor is only human. He or she may have expertise or a special interest in conditions other than endometriosis. It will help enormously if you can give accurate information and are clear and polite about what you want to say.

Tests for Endometriosis

The best way to diagnose endometriosis is to actually *see* it using a laparoscope. However, there are other tests that you might undergo before being referred for a laparoscopy, each described below.

Physical Examination

During a physical examination the doctor is looking for indications of possible endometriosis, such a pelvic mass (where organs feel as though they are matted together with scar tissue) that may feel tender, or, in the case of adenomyosis or fibroids, tissue that may make the uterus feel bulky. A physical examination may include:

- Feeling your abdomen on the outside to see if there is any tenderness, or if lumps can be felt through the abdominal wall muscles.

- Doing an internal examination to check that the vagina, uterus and ovaries aren't tender or affected by lumps.

- Examining the rectum to check the ligaments (muscle bands of strong tissue) and to see if there are any lumps behind the uterus.

But it is important to remember that if the outcome of any of these examinations is that everything seems normal, this doesn't mean that you don't have endometriosis. You may also be asked to come back another time because some problems don't show up until midcycle or just before or during your period.

Imaging Techniques

The *ultrasound scan* is the main imaging technique used to detect endometriosis. It is completely harmless and is the same device used to scan pregnant women. Some gel is put on to your stomach and a scanning head is then passed over your abdomen. It works by passing high-frequency sound waves through the body that then bounce back to form an image of your pelvic organs on a computer screen. The drawback with this method of diagnosis is that it can't distinguish between the different types of pelvic mass detected (that is, whether it has found an endometrial deposit, a cyst or a tumor). Another problem is that the scan generally only shows up deposits of over two centimeters in size. It can be of some help, though, in detecting whether the bowel or bladder is involved.

Other Investigations

The Bowel

If your bowel is thought to be affected by endometriosis, you may have the following tests:

- *Digital rectal examination:* Using a lubricated glove, a doctor examines the uterine ligaments using a finger and feels for lesions in the lower rectum. It is not usually painful, but can be a bit uncomfortable.

- *Barium enema:* During this procedure the lower bowel is filled with fluid via a tube inserted into the lower colon through the rectum. This fluid is made of a substance that shows up on X-rays and reveals areas where there are any constrictions or unusual growths.

- *Flexible sigmoidoscopy:* A narrow fiber-optic tube is passed into the lower bowel via the rectum. It allows the doctor to view the inner surface of the large bowel and to detect lesions. No anesthetic is necessary, but it may feel a bit uncomfortable.

Megan had a digital rectal examination after being referred to a bowel specialist because she was suffering continual diarrhea: "I was asked to undress from the waist down while the doctor left the room, and then to lie on my side on the bed with my knees up and my bottom exposed. He then came in and explained that he would be lubricating his finger and inserting it into my anus. Fortunately it didn't hurt; it just felt a bit uncomfortable. But it was all over very quickly and then he wiped the anus with a swab and gave me some disposable towels to clean away the lubrication."

Karen, a 31-year-old hospital support worker, had to undergo a barium enema before endometriosis was diagnosed. She recalls: "I was first given a muscle relaxant injection into my vein that was supposed to slow down the gut and stop the bowel from making spasms. It made me feel giddy and a bit sick. Then I had to lie on a table and a tube was inserted into my anus and up into my lower bowel. Air, and then fluid, was pumped into me via this thin tube. It did hurt quite a bit, but the medical staff treated me very well. I had to move around in different positions while they did the X-rays. Afterward it took me a couple of days to recover from feeling bruised and gassy!"

The Urinary Tract

These investigations include:

- *Kidney function tests:* To measure the amount of urea and salts in the blood, which can reveal whether your urinary system is involved.

- *Urinalysis:* A dip-stick test in a urine sample to exclude infection, kidney problems and diabetes as well as to detect urinary problems.

- *Urine microscopy:* A sample of urine is examined under a microscope for evidence of endometrial cells.

- *Urine culture:* Urine is observed to see if any bacteria grows in it, which could indicate an infection.

- *IVU (Intravenous Pyelogram):* An iodine-based solution is injected into an arm, enters the blood stream and is then X-rayed as it filters through the body to see if the kidney, ureter and bladder are functioning properly.

- *Cystoscopy:* A light anesthetic is given, and a viewing device called a *cystoscope* is inserted into the bladder to look for any lesions, which are then biopsied (that is, a small tissue sample is taken for laboratory analysis). This is sometimes done during routine laparoscopy.

- *Hysteroscopy:* Under local or general anesthetic, a tiny camera is inserted into the uterus vaginally to examine the lining.

Other Blood Tests

A sample of blood may be taken to look for evidence of infection or anemia, or for evidence of inflammation or disease.

Future Tests

Studies are still being carried out to develop a foolproof blood test that would reveal whether a woman has endometriosis. It has already been discovered that women with endometriosis have a raised amount of a substance called *CA125* in their blood, which is secreted by endometrial tissue. The problem is that this substance is also secreted in other women (such as those who are pregnant or have ovarian cancer), making it is impossible to tell without further investigation which condition is causing the rise in CA125.

Laparoscopy—The Primary Test for Endometriosis

What Is a Laparoscopy?

A *laparoscopy* is an operation to discover whether endometriosis is present in the pelvis. It involves having a *laparoscope*, a small telescope-like device, inserted through a small hole into your abdomen in order for the surgeon to see your insides. In some cases, the laparoscopy is used not only to diagnose endometriosis but also to perform surgery to remove any endometriosis found (see Chapter 9 for more on surgery and Chapter 10 on hysterectomy).

What Happens During a Laparoscopy?

The length of time you spend in hospital varies. Some hospitals do the surgery on an outpatient basis (for example, your surgery takes less than a day and you can go home afterward), whereas others may admit you for one or two nights.

A light general anesthetic will be given to put you to sleep throughout the operation. You will not be allowed to eat or drink for 12 hours before the operation, to avoid your vomiting during the surgery, which could be dangerous or even fatal.

Once you are under anesthetic, you are taken to the operating room where carbon dioxide gas is pumped via a small needle into your abdomen. This helps to separate your pelvic organs from each other—particularly your uterus and ovaries—making it easier for the surgeon to look for signs of endometriosis.

A small incision (cut) is then made near your navel to insert the laparoscope. Another small incision may be made above your pubic bone through which the surgeon's other instruments, such as a probe or biopsy forceps, can be passed, enabling him or her to look around properly. (Some surgeons use only the first hole for the whole operation, passing both the laparoscope and surgical instruments through it.) A probe is a thin rod of pliable metal with a blunt, swollen end used for exploring cavities without causing abrasions. Biopsy forceps are metal pincers used to extract tiny pieces of tissue for a laboratory examination.

While this is going on, the surgeon's assistant inserts a probe into your vagina, and passes it through your cervix and up into the uterus to help the surgeon manipulate the uterus in order to see more easily.

Any adhesions that are found are divided, both to allow the surgeon to see better and to relieve symptoms. This is usually done with scissors, or a heated cutting device in a process called *diathermy* or by a laser.

The operating table is then gently tipped to allow the coils of the bowel to slip down, making it easier for the surgeon to inspect the following areas:

- Ovaries

- Uterine wall

- Uterine ligaments

- Pouch of Douglas (the area behind the uterus)

- Colon and rectum (the colon is the main part of the large intestine, which, as part of the digestive process, removes nonabsorbed residue, and the rectum is the end of the large intestine where feces are stored)

- Ovarian ligaments

- Bladder surface

- Tubes running from the kidney to the bladder

Any cysts that are found during a laparoscopy are drained and biopsy samples are taken and sent for histology. A biopsy is the removal of small pieces of tissue. Histology is a microscopic examination of the biopsied tissue, using staining techniques to identify what kinds of cells they are, including endometrial cells. Some peritoneal fluid may also be drained and then analyzed as an aid to diagnosis.

Finally, the carbon dioxide gas is let out, the table is returned to the horizontal position and the small incisions are either stitched or stapled shut. The stitch may either dissolve or be removed by your physician.

After the Operation

You may need to take painkillers afterward because of the abdominal discomfort caused by the carbon dioxide gas. There may also be some vaginal bleeding, so sanitary napkins are usually advised, as they reduce the risk of infection that sometimes occurs after an operation that tampons could contribute to. Some women experience nausea and tiredness from the anesthetic. Many women also complain of shooting shoulder pains afterward, which are caused by the small amounts of carbon dioxide that are left behind that collect under the diaphragm (the sheet of muscle between the abdomen and the chest), causing referred pain (that is, pain experienced in a part of the body other than the site where it is produced) in your shoulders.

Estimated Recovery Time

Doctors usually advise taking up to a week off of work or home chores, but it is up to the individual concerned. Some women need more time, some less.

> Maria recalls, "I was given an information sheet that advised taking about three days off work. It also gave me the impression that I would get better very quickly.
>
> "Fortunately, I'd had arranged for a friend to meet me in her car because I would never have gotten home without her. I felt stiff and uncomfortable, and could hardly walk. Once at home, I went straight to bed and slept for 24 hours. Luckily my friend stayed with me and was able to cook my meals. But really, it

took me more than a week to recover. So I think it's important to be well prepared!"

Danger Signs

On occasion you can become ill after a laparoscopy if your pelvic organs have been accidentally damaged. You should contact your doctor immediately if you experience any of the following:

- Problems going to the bathroom
- Smelly vaginal discharge or heavy bleeding
- Feeling sick and vomiting
- Fever or chills
- Severe pain or increasing pain
- Redness or swelling around the wounds

What Are the Advantages of a Laparoscopy?

- It's the only definitive way to diagnose endometriosis, or to discover whether the cause of the discomfort you are experiencing is something else, like PID (see Chapter 3).
- The diagnosis is accurate in 70 percent of the investigations.
- Only small incisions are needed, making recovery fairly quick and reducing possible complications.

What Are the Disadvantages?

- The surgeon has to be highly trained and experienced to be able to use the instruments effectively.
- It can trigger internal adhesions.
- Endometriosis can't always be detected by the human eye.

- It's not always possible to treat extensive problems with this method, so a laparotomy may be required (see Chapter 9).

Take Note!

If you have a negative laparoscopy and the pain persists, it might be a good idea to press your doctor for a second laparoscopy.

"I Had a Laparoscopy"

Kim says, "I've had five laparoscopies and have found that every surgeon has a slightly different procedure. For instance, sometimes I've stayed in the hospital overnight and at other times I've just been a day-patient.

"Sometimes I've been asked to bathe and shave my pubic hair before the surgery—but not always. Often I go in early in the morning, so I stop eating and drinking at midnight the previous night. There can be quite a lot of waiting around in the hospital, so I take my personal CD player and a relaxation tape or two to calm my nerves.

"After having my chest listened to, and being asked such questions as whether I've had operations before, I change into a surgical gown. Sometimes I'm given a premedication, which make me feel woozy. At other times I'm immediately given the anesthetic. The surgeon usually says a few reassuring words before I go into the operating room.

"After the operation, the surgeon immediately tells me what he has found. Because it's sometimes difficult to ask all the questions I want at this stage, I sometimes write them down—just the basics, like what did they find? what treatment do they suggest? And so on.

"Generally, I recover quite easily and go back to work within a week. I don't get any abdominal pain at all, just a terrible shoulder ache, which is very common; I take an over-the-counter painkiller to relieve it. When I find myself able to do household tasks like the ironing without getting tired, I know I'm back to normal."

Classification of Endometriosis

There are various systems used to classify the different degrees of endometriosis, all of which calculate its severity according to a point system related to its internal distribution. The drawback with all of them is that they give points according to how far the disease is likely to affect your fertility—but they don't take into account other considerations, like how much pain you are experiencing. Apparently there is a new scale being developed that does take these things into account, but this scale hasn't come to fruition yet.

The most common classification system still used now is the one developed by the American Fertility Society (now called the American Society for Reproductive Medicine) in 1978, which was revised in 1985. Using this system, surgeons looks for lesions, nodules and cysts, giving points for each one found in specific areas and for their size. Adhesions are also counted on a rising scale, depending on their nature—that is, whether they are light or dense and whether they press into nearby healthy tissue. The extent of endometriosis is then usually described as minimal, mild, moderate or severe. Here are some examples of what this could mean:

> *Minimal* (Stage I): Superficial endometriosis on the peritoneum (the lining of the abdominal cavity) and filmy adhesions on one ovary

> *Mild* (Stage II): Shallow implants on the pelvic lining and on one ovary, with filmy adhesions on the other ovary

> *Moderate* (Stage III): Deep deposits on the pelvic lining and on one ovary, dense adhesions on the other ovary

> *Severe* (Stage IV): Deep deposits on the ovaries, with dense adhesions on the ovary, fallopian tube and pelvic lining

The patches of endometriosis seen through the laparoscope vary greatly in appearance and are commonly described in a number of ways:

- Classic, gun-metal–blue-gray spots
- "Raspberry" spots, with shaggy tissue at the edges
- Flat or raised white tissue, like scarring
- Clear "berries" with small peaks
- "Chocolate" cysts filled with old blood

These endometriosis deposits can be further classified according to the nature of their cells. The uterine lining normally has three different types of cells:

- Surface cells
- Glands
- *Stroma* (the connective tissue that binds the glands together)

The more deeply embedded these cells are, the more difficult they are to remove. They can also be further graded according to their level of activity. Early, active cells usually have no color, but when tested in the laboratory often have more biochemical activity than the older, darker colored areas of endometriosis, which can mean that they are more painful.

Take Note!

The main thing to remember is that, although your endometriosis may have been classified as mild, it may not *feel* mild; and it needs to be taken just as seriously as a case of severe endometriosis that causes little pain.

CHAPTER FIVE

Infertility

Infertility and Endometriosis

Infertility is an inability to conceive. It is important to remember that women with endometriosis are not necessarily sterile. However, it sometimes takes longer for them to get pregnant. They are therefore often referred to as "subfertile" rather than infertile. Strictly speaking, you can be diagnosed as subfertile if you have failed to conceive after 12 months of regular, unprotected intercourse.

How Many Women Are Affected?

Various studies suggest that 30 to 50 percent of women with endometriosis are infertile, and that endometriosis is the cause of infertility in 30 percent of all infertile women. Some researchers take this to mean that there is a link between the two, although the nature of the link is still unknown. What *is* known, however, is that infertility becomes more likely as the disease progresses. This is one of the reasons that women should be treated for endometriosis as soon as they are diagnosed. But it is usually only women with severe cases of the disease who may have difficulty conceiving as a result of their endometriosis.

How Could Endometriosis Affect My Fertility?

As we have said, the reasons aren't really known, but some side effects of endometriosis—such as damage to the ovaries and fallopian tubes, adhesions and scar tissue (resulting from the disease or from surgery), irregular periods, pain with sex and possible hormonal factors may contribute to infertility The more severe the endometriosis, the more likely it is to cause an infertility problem.

Two types of infertility are usually associated with endometriosis:

Endometrial deposits: These may secrete substances that somehow interfere with pregnancy.

Pelvic damage: Some women suffering from endometriosis have ovaries distorted by large "chocolate" cysts; or the finger-like ends of their fallopian tubes may be distorted by lesions or blocked by adhesions.

Other Theories

SPERM AND EGG TRANSPORT

One theory has it that hormonelike chemicals called prostaglandins (see Chapter 1), which are produced by areas of endometriosis, enter the fallopian tubes and affect the transport of the sperm and/or the egg in a way that reduces the chances of conceiving.

OVARIAN DYSFUNCTION

This theory is based on research that shows that some women with endometriosis don't always release an egg during their menstrual cycle. However, it's difficult to say whether this is caused solely by endometriosis, because it also happens to women who *don't* have endometriosis.

UNRUPTURED FOLLICLE SYNDROME

Some researchers believe that in certain women with endometriosis, ripe eggs sometimes don't hatch from their follicles, but instead stay trapped inside. However, other findings suggest that this is no more likely to happen in endometriosis sufferers than in any other women.

IMMUNOLOGY

It is thought that women with endometriosis have some abnormalities in their immune system (see Chapter 3), and that this might play a role in stopping a fertilized egg from implanting in the uterus. It's still not clear whether this is the case, but research is continuing.

PROLACTIN LEVELS

The hormone *prolactin* is usually secreted during pregnancy, but is sometimes produced outside pregnancy if the pituitary gland grows too big. Too much prolactin is thought to inhibit fertility. Levels are usually checked routinely in women who suffer from subfertility, and a drug called bromocriptine is prescribed, which lowers prolactin secretion.

PERITONEAL FLUID

This fluid is found in the peritoneum (the fluid membrane that lines the abdominal cavity, encasing all the organs). Scavenger cells are usually present in this fluid to mop up bacteria and endometrial blood, and to stop sperm from swimming out of the fallopian tubes. Infertile women with endometriosis seem to have a higher number of these scavengers, which could block the movement of the sperm and the egg along the tubes, or even affect the implantation of an embryo.

RECURRENT MISCARRIAGE

Miscarriage is defined as the failure of pregnancy before Week 24, and *recurrent miscarriage* is if it happens more than twice. (After 24 weeks the loss is termed a *stillbirth*.) Some early studies show that miscarriage is three times as common in women with endometriosis (mostly within the first 12 weeks of pregnancy). However, other studies indicate that this could have more to do with the woman's previous obstetric history than the presence of endometriosis.

What Is the Best Treatment For Infertility and Endometriosis?

It's important to get treatment for endometriosis as soon as possible, because it does sometimes worsen over time. However, because the available treatments are usually only temporary, and because all the treatments entail certain risks, women with mild endometriosis may be advised to follow a wait-and-see approach, that is, trying for a pregnancy for 6 to 12 months before embarking on treatment. It has been found that during that time 20 percent of the women are likely to conceive. After waiting, drug treatment is usually prescribed if the disease has progressed, and then if problems still remain, assisted conception techniques may be suggested.

Take Note!

It isn't always a good idea to embark immediately on stressful in vitro fertilization *(IVF)* treatment. The important thing to remember is that lots of women with endometriosis *do* get pregnant. The first things to do are to make sure that you are fit and well, and that your immune system is healthy.

Drug Treatment for Infertile Endometriosis Sufferers

If the endometriosis deposits aren't too deep, contraceptive pills may at first be suggested as a way of buying time until you feel ready to have a baby. More severe drug treatments such as danazol, progestogens and GnRH analogues (see Chapter 8) may be suggested if the Pill does not work.

There are certain warnings about using the noncontraceptive drug treatments for women who want to conceive. If you become pregnant while on hormone therapy, there is a chance that the baby may be deformed. Therefore treatment is always started when you are sure you aren't pregnant. Also, some women still ovulate when on the treatment, so it is advisable to use barrier methods of contraception while undergoing drug treatment.

Furthermore, pregnancy shouldn't be attempted until after you've had a normal period after the treatment has been stopped. This allows the body time to readjust. Also, progesterone treatment is not a good option for women considering pregnancy soon, because it can suppress ovulation for quite a while after the treatment has finished—sometimes for up to a year.

How Successful Is Drug Treatment?

Pregnancy rate statistics aren't reliable yet for the pregnancy rate of endometriosis sufferers following treatment. With the Pill, estimates range from 5 to 75 percent. Such varying statistics exist for danazol as well. But what *is* known is that it is easier to conceive in the early months following treatment rather than the later months, because you are more free from endometriosis. The longer you wait, the more likely it is that endometriosis will reappear.

Surgery

Depending on the degree of endometriosis, reconstruction can be done with a laparotomy or using a laparoscopy and lasers. Endometrial deposits can be cut or burned away, any adhesions and damaged ovaries or tubes removed, and organs restored to their correct positions. Some reports indicate that laser surgery conserves fertility better because less tissue is destroyed and scar tissue doesn't result. However, there are no reliable figures on this.

Surgery is definitely a good option if you have large cysts or extensive problems that are not easily treatable with drugs. If you are older, you might also feel that you don't have enough time for the wait-and-see approach, or for drug treatment, which takes at least six months.

Disadvantages of Surgery

One disadvantage of surgery is that it might lead to more adhesions, which could contribute further to infertility. It's sometimes thought best to use a combination of surgery and drug treatment because it's impossible to remove all endometrial sites with surgery alone: the surgeon can't see microscopic patches of endometriosis or treat endometriosis in sensitive areas such as on the organs (see Chapter 9).

How Successful Is Surgery?

With conservative surgery during a laparotomy, the pregnancy rate is 75 percent in mild cases, 65 percent in moderate cases and 50 percent in severe cases. Other reports on success rates after surgery range from about 38 to 88 percent, so the results are somewhat unreliable again. However, what is known is that the success afterward depends on the extent of the disease before the treatment.

Will the Baby Be Healthy?

Yes—although unfortunately, women with endometriosis have a slightly higher rate of miscarriage and ectopic pregnancy (that is, the fetus develops outside the uterus). The higher rate of ectopic pregnancy is probably due to fallopian tube damage. The danger signs for an ectopic pregnancy are a slight bleeding 7 to 14 days after a missed period, mild soreness or pain that gets sharper later, and fainting and nausea. Help should be sought immediately as an ectopic pregnancy is potentially life threatening, because it can cause the fallopian tube to rupture, resulting in serious internal bleeding.

Fertility Treatments

After your endometriosis has been treated, you may go on to have fertility treatment if you haven't yet become pregnant. This may entail the following procedures and tests.

Sex During Your Fertile Stage

A lot of people are unaware that there is a relatively short time each month when a woman can get pregnant. It is only 48 hours after ovulation, that is, the release of an egg. If your cycle is 28 days, this will usually be Day 14 (if Day 1 is the start of your period). But actually there are seven days when you can conceive, because the sperm can survive for about five days inside a woman's body waiting for the egg. So five days before the egg is released and two days after the egg is released are your most fertile times. Simply buying an ovulation prediction kit that measures the hormones in your urine may help you become pregnant.

Keeping Temperature Charts

A woman is often asked to keep a temperature chart, because this gives doctors a clue as to whether she is releasing any eggs at all. A woman's central body temperature usually goes up by a fraction of a degree when she ovulates. However, because you have to take your temperature first thing and record it every day, this is sometimes thought to put undue stress on some women (an ovulation kit, as mentioned above, might be better).

Undergoing Infertility Tests

Blood tests: These are usually done on Day 21 of your cycle. They test the levels of the various reproductive hormones in your bloodstream (progesterone is thought to be at its highest when you have ovulated). Your partner may also take a semen test for analysis at the same time.

Postcoital tests: If the blood and semen tests prove inconclusive, you may have a postcoital test whereby mucus from your cervix is sent for analysis after sex. If live, active sperm are seen, then the test is normal.

If there are problems with either of these, further tests may follow:

- ◆ Ultrasound scan
- ◆ Fallopian tube testing
- ◆ Laparoscopy
- ◆ Falloscopy (a flexible telescope inserted into the fallopian tubes to make sure they aren't scarred or blocked or to clear debris from their ends)
- ◆ Other sperm tests

Taking Fertility Drugs

Your doctor may suggest taking a fertility drug like Clomid (Clomid and Serophene are both trade names for clomiphene citrate). This drug is used to treat ovulation failure and works by simulating the ovaries into producing several mature eggs at the same time.

Using Assisted Conception Techniques

What Is In Vitro Fertilization (IVF)?

In vitro fertilization is normally used in conjunction with a fertility drug like Clomid. The patient is then monitored with ultrasound equipment to find out when one of the ovary sacs will burst open. As the time approaches, a fine needle is passed through the wall of the abdomen to suck out some of these ripe eggs, which are then mixed with the partner's sperm. Once fertilization has taken place, they may be put directly into the uterus at some stage.

> Helen, a 35-year-old accountant, started IVF after a laparoscopy revealed she had mild endometriosis that could be interfering with one of her fallopian tubes.
>
> "I was put on drug therapy first for six months," she comments, "which sometimes gave me terrible hot flashes and quite painful breasts, but which seemed to make my usual PMS symptoms disappear completely. Then I was told I could have IVF treatment immediately, or wait three months and then try. My physician explained that during my laparoscopy they had flushed out my fallopian tubes and that I might want to see whether that had worked, first of all. But I decided to go straight for IVF instead. First, my husband and I went to have basic tests such as a scan to check that my ovaries were working properly, and I had a Day 21 progesterone blood test to make sure that my hormones were also working. I had a vaginal swab taken to rule out infections such as PID.
>
> "Then I was given a nasal spray, which I had to take every four hours. Apparently, if you take this drug first, your ovaries

are more likely to respond to the fertility drugs. I found it horrendous trying to remember it all the time, and had to carry a little alarm clock around with me. I was quite worried because they said that if I took it just ten minutes late it would mean that my female hormone levels would go back up.

"They then scanned me to see whether my ovaries were in a state to start taking fertility drugs. I started on the Pergonol injections (a fertility drug) on a Friday, and was given an injection every day and scanned each day to see how my eggs were developing. They have to be careful not to overstimulate you because this can be dangerous.

"The following Friday, they looked to see whether I'd produced enough eggs for them to operate. I had. Then, ten days later, I was taken into the operating room; the eggs were extracted and then fertilized with my husband's sperm in a test tube. Two days later I went back again and the eggs were inserted into me very simply via a catheter (it's just like having a smear). Then we had to wait for two weeks to see if I was pregnant.

"I had this procedure done twice unsuccessfully, but then I started going to stress management classes run by my HMO for women with fertility problems. I learned how to breathe properly and to do self-hypnosis and was encouraged to talk about any worries that might be blocking me from becoming pregnant. For instance, I realized that I was very anxious about money problems if I became pregnant, although I didn't really need to be. Within three months (in between IVF attempts) I got pregnant naturally. Now I'm about to give birth. I can't tell what helped me conceive—all I can say is that I'm delighted!"

What Is GIFT?

GIFT stands for *Gamete Intra-Fallopian Transfer,* and means that the gametes (the sperm and egg) are put back into the uterus at an earlier stage than in ordinary IVF treatment. They are usually flushed into the fallopian tubes, where fertilization may be more likely to take place because of the more natural environment. This procedure is not as common as IVF.

Are There Any Alternative Treatments?

Vitamin E, zinc and the herbal extract vitex agnus castus are said to improve fertility; treatments such as acupuncture for the pain, chiropractic and homeopathy have also been found to be beneficial. Nutrition and exercise may also help. For instance, a high-protein diet and B vitamins are thought to be especially important (see Chapter 6).

Should I Keep Trying?

Paula says, "When I was told that I had virtually no chance of conceiving because of endometriosis and because my husband's sperm count was low, we decided we didn't really mind not being able to have children. We both have fulfilling careers and we didn't want to go through the trauma of in vitro fertilization. After a course of danazol, we stopped using contraceptives, but within two years I was surprised and delighted to find I was pregnant. We were advised after that to try quickly again if we wanted any more children, and just 16 months later our next one came along. So I can't help thinking if you're relaxed about pregnancy it is more likely to happen."

Joanne's experiences were very different: "I've decided that, although I'm only 27, I'd like to have a hysterectomy. Trying to have a baby has made me feel suicidal. I just can't cope with my hopes constantly being dashed. Between us, my husband and I have decided that my quality of life and our being happy together is more important than a baby. I want to put it all behind me and get on with my life. And I realize, too, that now that the pressure is off, I wasn't quite as bothered about it as I thought I was. Talking about it in the endometriosis support groups in my community has really helped me come to this decision."

Is Pregnancy a Cure for Endometriosis?

Doctors have long believed that pregnancy is a cure for endometriosis. It *is* true, insofar as pregnancy can help endometrial deposits clear up, because your periods stop for nine months. However, although many women do report a lessening of their symptoms during pregnancy, they often say endometriosis returns afterward—and the more severe the case is, the more severely it usually returns.

If you feel better during pregnancy, a way to lengthen the time of remission is to breastfeed, since ovulation is believed to be suppressed by breastfeeding. However, there have been some reports to the American Endometriosis Association that the disease worsens during pregnancy, although no studies have yet been done on this.

Having said that, even if you want to take your chances and see if it works for you, you should still carefully consider whether you really want a baby at this point in your life.

Points to consider:

1. Don't rush into it.

2. Talk to women from your local endometriosis support group who are in a similar situation.

3. Speak to a counselor or therapist sensitive to your situation to help you sort out your feelings.

Moving Toward a Natural Approach

In this and the previous four chapters, you have read about the symptoms and causes of endometriosis, as well as ways to test for and diagnose the disease. In Part II you will learn coping strategies such as diet modification, exercise, the use of food supplements and lifestyle changes, and you will discover a range of complementary therapies—ranging from acupuncture to yoga—that can help you find relief.

PART TWO
A Natural Approach

CHAPTER SIX

Coping Strategies

Coping with Your Pain

Learning to deal with the pain is important for endometriosis sufferers. Here are some practical tips on things that have helped other sufferers (in alphabetical order).

Baths and Relaxation

Many women find that encouraging muscles to relax, either through taking a bath or practicing a relaxation technique, can help menstrual pain considerably. Breathing deeply may also help; many HMOs offer classes on diaphragmatic breathing and biofeedback techniques.

Diet

Eating a sufficient, varied and good diet is particularly important during a menstrual period. Many women have also found that reducing salt (which aggravates PMS bloating), sugar (which can cause yeast problems), alcohol and caffeine intake (which make you feel more irritable and stressed) is beneficial during their periods. (There is more about diet later in this chapter.)

Exercise

One of the best measures for combating pain is exercise, which results in the body's producing its own natural painkillers. Bicycling, swimming, aerobics and fast walking are particularly useful. Exercise can also be helpful emotionally, if only to take your mind off your pain for a while.

If you find that even walking is too painful, you could try the following exercise instead:

1. Lie flat on the floor with a pillow behind your knees.

2. Beginning with your feet, work up your body, tensing your feet, calves, thighs, buttocks, and so on, all the way up to your neck and facial muscles.

3. Breathe in, hold each set of muscles tight for 5 to 10 seconds, and then let your breath out. It should take about ten minutes, and you should notice a result!

(There is more on exercise later in this chapter.)

Flotation Therapy

One form of therapy reported to be good for pain relief is flotation. You literally float on the top of a tank of water that contains a salt solution to stop you from sinking. It is also thought that the experience of floating alters the electrical activity in the brain, promoting profound relaxation.

Heat and Cold

Heating pads or hotwater bottles can reduce muscle spasms and increase the flow of blood. A sauna or warm bath can also have the same effect. Likewise, rubbing something cold such as package of frozen peas on the site of the pain until the skin feels numb can reduce pain.

Keeping a Pain Diary or Scrapbook

Many sufferers have found it useful to keep a simple diary of their pain, to help to take their mind off it and as a useful resource to show their physician.

> Christine says, "Keeping a diary helped me to put my frustrations down on paper and then to let go of them. I also showed it to my doctor, who said it was a great help to him to see my cyclical pattern."

> Elizabeth found that it helped to create a scrapbook. "I got the idea from one of the self-help books," she says. "I'm not an artsy person, but I got a scrapbook and gluestick and some crayons. I stuck in my favorite quotes from books I'd found useful, cartoons from the newspaper, a photo of myself and some information on drugs that my doctor had given me, and also names of vitamins I was taking. That particular self-help book also encouraged me to try and picture what my pain looks like and even draw it. It was very hard at first, but there is no right or wrong way of doing it. My drawings of colored blobs on scraps of paper (often done in five minutes at work) won't win any prizes, but they gave me a physical map of how I felt at that moment and this was very useful.

> "I also write down how I feel in my special book and give my pain a star rating. Five stars is the worst—that's when I find it hard just to put my stockings on in the morning. The scrapbook has really helped me continue working when I've been in great pain."

Massage

Forms of massage can also be very helpful in coping with pain. Massage involves a variety of rubbing and kneading techniques that help to relieve tension, improve circulation and reduce pain and high blood pressure. You can see a qualified practitioner, get (or trade) a full-body massage from a loved one or partner, or try the following self-help techniques yourself:

For menstrual pain: Using a V-stroke from one hipbone down to the pubic hairline and up to the other hipbone, firmly apply your fingertips in a circular direction just above the pubic hairline.

For ovulation pain: Apply the massage in a circular motion just below the inside anklebone.

For back pain: Massage the bottom of your feet along the inside arch, or roll your bare foot back and forth over a ribbed cola bottle or a special massage tool.

Orgasm

Having an orgasm can be good for menstrual pain, as it naturally causes the uterus to contract and helps to expel blood.

Pain Management

There are many pain management centers throughout the country that your doctor may be able to refer you to. The following are just a few:

The American Chronic Pain Association, P.O. Box 850, Rocklin, CA 95677; 916-632-0922.

The American Pain Society, 4700 West Lake Avenue, Glenview, IL 60025; 847-375-4715.

The Commission for the Accreditation of Rehabilitation Facilities (CARF), 4891 East Grant Road, Tucson, AZ 95712; 520-325-1044.

TEN TIPS ON COPING WITH PAIN

Jan Sadler, a member of Painwise UK (England), gives the following advice on how to cope with a flare-up of pain:

1. *Stay positive:* The most important thing you can do is to decide to take charge of the situation by facing and

accepting it. Accept that it has happened and that there is nothing to be gained by blaming anyone, especially yourself. A really helpful phrase to say to yourself is, "Be still—this will pass."

2. *Plan:* Try not to let yourself get so overwhelmed that you abandon all the helpful strategies that you have learned in the past. Write a list, and mentally decide which techniques you need at the moment.

3. *Relax:* At least once a day, take time for a 15- to 20-minute deep relaxation session. Find a quiet place and use whatever method suits you. One of the simplest methods employed in meditation is to "watch" your breath as it goes in and out, and as your mind wanders gently bring it back to your breath again.

4. *Use affirmations:* This is simply repeating a few special words that reflect how you would like to be, such as "I am peaceful and calm" or "Day by day I am getting better and better." Make up some useful ones that you can write on little cards to refer to when you need them.

5. *Visualization:* Spend some time creating pictures in your mind. Imagine yourself floating in a hot-air balloon, or visualize changing your pain into something more comfortable. For example, burning pains could be cooled by imagining yourself standing under a waterfall on a tropical island.

6. *Pace yourself:* Cut down your sitting, standing and walking times to a level you can cope with—even if it's only half a minute at a time. Then get a timer (or a sports watch with a timer) and start a pacing program. Set your timer to the number of minutes you've decided to spend on each activity, and when it rings change tasks. Very slowly increase these times.

7. *Keep your body active:* Exercise is very important, even if you are just starting with stretching your fingers

and toes. Make a start and then space the exercises out throughout the day. Swimming is particularly good because the water is supportive, preventing the dragging pain you may feel when walking.

8. *Keep your mind active:* Try to keep to your daily routine as much as possible. Even if it's just reading a book, watching TV or surfing the Internet, it can help distract you.

9. *Use helping aids:* Try some of the other pain relief methods mentioned in this book, such as aromatherapy or acupuncture.

10. *Be patient:* That means living in the here and now, not with one foot planted in next week. In yearning for the future the whole time, we miss everything around us and simply create more tension for ourselves. Be kind to yourself and focus on what you can do this moment—and not what you can't!

For more information see Jan Sadler's book, *Natural Pain Relief*, listed in "Further Reading" at the back of this book.

Pelvic Exercises

Pelvic congestion before periods can be relieved by pelvic exercises (also known as Kegels) that tone up the pelvic floor muscles, stimulate circulation in the area and help drain away any excess fluid.

To find out which are your pelvic muscles, try stopping the urine flow the next time you go to the bathroom—the muscles you naturally find yourself using are your pelvic floor muscles. If you can stop the flow instantly, your muscles are in good shape. If you can't, try the following exercise:

1. Lie flat on your back with your knees bent and your feet flat on the floor.

2. Imagine pulling something in and up into your vagina. You'll probably find yourself tightening your

buttocks as you do this, but make sure these aren't the only muscles you're tightening.

3. Hold the muscles for a slow count of five and then release them.

4. You could test how well you are doing by holding your fingers in your vagina and trying to tighten the pelvic muscles around them.

TENS *(Transcutaneous Electrical Nerve Stimulation)*

This method of pain relief involves using a tiny electronic device that is smaller than a Walkman, which has two to four electrodes attached to it. The electrodes are placed on the body in the area of the pain, and then the machine is switched on, generating a tiny electrical impulse through the body. This stimulator can be used with good effects for anything from half-an-hour to eight hours a day. It works by stimulating endorphins in the body, which are our own natural painkillers.

You need a prescription in order to get one, and a physical therapist or physician must train you on how to use it. Check with your doctor. Prices range from $660 to $800.

Coping with Your Feelings

Depression

A lot of women with endometriosis are also depressed. As we've said already, it is hardly surprising that women suffering from endometriosis feel depressed when they are dealing with such a confusing, debilitating and little-understood illness. Women suffering from endometriosis often say the following things about endometriosis: "No one believes me!" Or "My friends don't understand why I'm in pain!" Or "Everyone thinks I'm a hypochondriac!"

If you feel like this, you might ask your doctor to refer you to a counselor so that you can speak to someone with a sympathetic ear. The main thing to remember is: you're not going crazy!

Jackie says, "I've had a few appointments with my counselor—really just to vent about the way I've been treated in the past year. I'd felt very angry that my continued pain was ignored, and that at one stage I was even sent to a psychiatrist because of it. I felt it was important to get over this. I then discussed my thoughts about the future, such as about my fertility and my relationship with my boyfriend. I've found counseling helpful because it has put things into perspective. It was also good to have someone acknowledging my feelings without blaming me for feeling the way I did."

Your Partner and Family

During one seminar on pain management, it became clear that one of the biggest problems for endometriosis sufferers was the guilt they felt about their partners and families. Sufferers often felt that because of the pain, they weren't able to be proper mothers or wives or partners.

If you are in this situation, you might find it helpful to take your spouse or partner to a coed session of a local endometriosis group. If there are no groups available, or he would not like that kind of thing, you could get him as well as other members of your family to read some of the literature on the subject so that they will understand exactly what you're going through.

Eleanor's partner, Nick, says, "When I knew more about the condition, it helped me to be more understanding. I could see why Eleanor was so frustrated by the lack of a correct diagnosis. It also made me realize that it was good for her to talk about it, since she had suffered a lot in silence in the past."

Jackie describes some of the difficulties endometriosis has caused in her relationship: "I met my partner just over two years ago and it has been a relationship of discovery for both of us. The endometriosis has made me—and consequently us—address issues earlier than we normally would. For instance, we've had to address the problem of painful sex. And it's been very difficult working out whether I'm tensing up because of the anticipated pain or whether sex is just painful in itself.

"Endometriosis can also be a difficult concept to put across: what it means, how it feels, the pain, the surgery options and the drug treatments available. But early on in our relationship I was quite open about it. If I felt really horrible on a given day, I couldn't lie about it or pretend the pain didn't exist, and would acknowledge it as a 'not-so-good day.'

"But fortunately my partner is loving and caring enough for endometriosis not to be a 'problem.' At times, I admit, I would test him to see how much my having endometriosis affected us, but he would just say that he couldn't separate the two. My not having endometriosis wouldn't necessarily make us any better, however much he wished I didn't have the pain—this thing unfortunately is part of me and he thinks I'm strong enough to handle it, and he loves me as a whole person.

"However, being in a relationship brings with it a new set of issues: Where do we go from here? Can I conceive a child? Do I want to conceive? Do I want to have a baby in this relationship? How much time do I have? How much time do I have between treatments? All those sorts of things!"

Coping with Sexual Problems

Lack of sex is a significant problem in the relationships of endometriosis sufferers. In one survey it was reported that 55 percent of sufferers experience painful sex. This can cause quite a strain between you and your partner, who may understandably feel very rejected. Talking is always the best option.

Tips on How to Make Sex Less Painful

Make sure you are fully aroused before penetration: it is less likely to cause pain because if you are properly lubricated. Full arousal (through ample and enjoyable foreplay) also causes the vagina to elongate and the cervix to move farther up so that you are less likely to brush sensitive areas such as the Pouch of Douglas or the pelvic organs. It also makes it less likely that your vagina muscles will close spontaneously.

If you have problems with a dry vagina (one of the menopausal symptoms that can result from drug treatment), try a lubricant such as KY jelly, other vaginal moisturizers or vitamin E oil rubbed into the vagina.

Also bear in mind that just because you don't have penetration it does not mean you're not having sex! You could try arousing each other in different ways and experimenting with other types of sex. A self-help manual may give you some ideas.

Take note: Pain with deep penetration during intercourse, or painful contractions during orgasm, can sometimes be a result of the uterine muscles' becoming sensitive during drug treatment.

What Does Counseling Do?

Thankfully, many different types of counseling are available today. Some involve in-depth psychotherapy that can go on for several years; others are short term and very goal orientated—that is, you come with a view to solving a very specific problem. What either type of therapy will do will be to help you explore your feelings about your illness and how it affects your relationships. But a good therapist will not tell you what to do—their purpose is to help you understand yourself better.

The thing to remember is that counseling is a positive step. More and more people seek counseling these days, and it certainly doesn't mean you are going crazy.

> Lisa says, "I saw a counselor at the college where I was a student many years ago. Although she wasn't as empathetic and warm as I'd hoped, she did help me come to terms with the anger I felt toward doctors. Having been misdiagnosed for 4 years and made to feel like a malingerer, I was understandably very upset. She helped me to be able to talk to doctors in a level voice, and to see that my anger against them was destructive for me. Sometimes when I'd finished a session I went away feeling I could put all those worries away, and for a moment it was as though I was walking on air!"

Self-Help Groups

Time and time again, endometriosis sufferers have said how much support groups have helped them. These groups do all sorts of things, from sharing their feelings, to giving advice on relaxation techniques; some even have sessions that include partners now and then. Some find it helpful in practical ways; others say that just sharing their feelings with others in the same boat makes them feel less isolated. If there isn't an endometriosis group in your area, you could try joining a general women's self-help group, or ask your HMO to consider forming such a group.

> Janet says, "When I first went to the endometriosis support group, I just cried and cried. Then they helped me write a letter to my physician putting down my experiences down on paper, clearly and simply. The letter helped me get a proper consultation with him and to be at last taken seriously. Also, the group helped me to fight to get my early retirement pension. It took 18 months, and in the end I had to settle on 'arthritis' as the cause, even though it was endometriosis. But the group's support still helped me not to give up and settle for less."

Dietary Advice

It is generally assumed that a basic healthy diet is good for endometriosis sufferers. The "rules" are simple:

- Eat plenty of vegetables and fresh fruit.
- Eat as many whole foods as possible, such as wholegrain cereals.
- Where possible, grill, steam or stew foods rather than fry them.
- Eat more foods rich in essential fatty acids, such as seeds, nuts and grains.
- Cook in oil rather than fat.
- Eat low-fat versions of dairy products (for example, non- or low-fat milk).

- Cut down on sugar (and remember that sugar is added to most processed foods, including frozen dinners and snack foods; read labels carefully).

- Reduce your intake of salt and animal fats.

- Choose white meats, such as chicken, rather than red meat.

- Drink less coffee, tea and carbonated drinks.

- Drink at least six glasses of water a day.

Don't expect to change your diet overnight. Try out new ideas as you go along, and transform your eating habits gradually—you might even find it exciting and beneficial in many ways.

Vitamin and Mineral Supplements

Some women have noticed an improvement in general health when taking an ordinary multivitamin and mineral tablet. If you don't want the hassle of taking a lot of different pills, you could try taking one for a few months to see if it improves your symptoms. Different brands vary considerably, so if you react negatively to one brand try another.

Alternatively, if you would like to go into it in more detail, find an alternative practitioner or holistic counselor who specializes in nutritional or vitamin therapies.

Evening Primrose Oil

One essence, Evening Primrose oil, is thought to be good for alleviating PMS and can also reduce the side effects of drug treatment (such as tiredness and water retention caused by danazol). This oil contains a substance called GLA (gamma linoleic acid), believed to enhance the production of a particular prostaglandin, which regulates several of the body functions involved in PMS.

Natural sources of GLA include cold-pressed safflower oil (available from health food stores). Starflower oil (sometimes called borage oil) is thought to contain three times as much GLA as Evening Primrose oil, but in a somewhat different chemical form. Further research is needed to assess its potential.

Suggested daily intake: two to three 500 mg. tablets for general health; four to six 500 mg. tablets for PMS.

> Suzanne, who had a cyst removed from her right ovary, says, "Primrose oil has definitely eased my pain a great deal. I find if I just stop it for one day, I begin to get pains down the back of my legs."

Dolomite (Calcium/Magnesium)

Calcium and magnesium improve muscle tone that makes the contractions during your period more even and less painful. Calcium absorption may be reduced if your magnesium intake is too low, so they are usually taken together. For still better absorption, take calcium (*not* Tums or other antacids, which are mostly sugar) with low doses of vitamins D and E. Vitamin E improves the healing of scar tissue caused by internal endometrial bleeding. However, as dolomite is not absorbed easily, other sources of calcium and magnesium may be better.

Magnesium sources: Green, leafy vegetables; grapefruit, figs, apples, nuts and seeds.

Calcium sources: Dried beans, green vegetables, peanuts, walnuts, sunflower seeds, sardines.

Daily intake: 200–800 mg.

Vitamin B_6 (Pyridoxine)

Vitamin B_6 reduces symptoms of PMS, such as depression, bloating, headaches and breast tenderness. It particularly seems to help endometriosis sufferers who experience these symptoms for the entire month. It's a good idea to take it with vitamin B complex for a balanced intake. (Be careful not to overdose on B vitamins, since that can lead to nerve damage.)

Vitamin B_6 also helps with the side effects of such hormone treatments as danazol, especially the tiredness and depression it can cause.

Natural sources: Brewer's yeast (avoid this if you're sensitive to yeast), wheat germ, cabbage, eggs.

Suggested daily intake: 100 mg. (50 mg. twice a day), together with 25 to 50 mg. of vitamin B complex (depending on the strength).

Vitamin E

It's important that endometriosis sufferers get enough Vitamin E, because it keeps scar tissue soft and flexible, reducing the pain caused by adhesions. It is best to start with 100 IU (international units) twice daily and to increase gradually.

Take note: Check with your physician if you have blood pressure problems. Anyone with high blood pressure should not exceed 400 IU daily without medical supervision. Anyone on anticoagulant therapy should also avoid vitamin E unless under medical supervision.

Natural sources: Green vegetables, wholegrain cereal, soy beans, eggs.

Daily intake: from 200 to 600 IU, to be increased gradually.

Vitamin C

Extra vitamin C can help if you suffer from heavy bleeding, because it strengthens blood vessel walls and aids in the absorption of iron (which helps make red blood cells). It can also help you heal after surgery, and some endometriosis sufferers have reported that it is good for pain. It also helps strengthen the immune system.

Natural sources: Green vegetables, potatoes, citrus fruits, black currants.

Daily intake: 500 mg. to 1 g.

Vitamin D

The D vitamin is important for calcium absorption and helps bone formation. Do not take a higher dose than recommended; too much Vitamin D is toxic.

Natural sources: Fatty fish, eggs.

Daily intake: 350–400 IU

Selenium

This trace element is taken together with vitamins A, C and E. It is available in several forms, some of which have a yeast base that is thought to improve the absorption of selenium. (If you have yeast or *candida* problems, check the label to make sure you buy one *without* yeast.) Selenium and vitamin E are supposed to give protection to the body, producing an anti-inflammatory effect. Selenium is also known to strengthen the immune system, which, as we know, is an important factor in fighting endometriosis.

Natural sources: Garlic, broccoli, tomatoes, wheat germ, tuna.

Daily intake: 1 tablet, 200 mcg.

Zinc

Another mineral, zinc, is thought to help in the treatment of PMS by countering depression; it also promotes healing and fertility.

Natural sources: Eggs, oysters, herring, wheat germ, seeds, nuts.

Daily intake: 10–30 mg.

Supplement Dos and Don'ts

- Don't take isolated vitamins or minerals without the advice of a qualified practitioner.

- Generally, it is best to take supplements with meals because they are more easily absorbed. However, there are some exceptions, such as zinc, which is thought to be absorbed better at night on an empty stomach.

- When buying a multivitamin supplement, do opt for one with a wide and balanced variety of minerals and vitamins.

- Don't be tempted to take supplements instead of eating balanced meals.

- Don't take huge doses of vitamins and supplements.

More Specific Diet Guidelines

Some sufferers have found the following specific dietary treatments helpful.

The Natural Estrogen Diet

Some researchers believe that by eating foods containing weak plant estrogens (*isoflavonoids*), you may actually be able to reduce the amount of estrogen in your own body. However, the idea is very controversial and the benefits haven't yet been fully substantiated.

Foods that are a rich source of these include:

- Dried fruits

- Cabbages and turnips

- Berries, peas and legumes

- Beans, nuts and seeds

- Unrefined grain products, such as rye products

- Soy products such as tofu and soy milk

- It isn't advisable to change your diet radically without detailed advice and supervision from a physician, alternative practitioner or nutritionist.

Extra Vitamins C, E and Beta-carotene

A diet rich in vitamins C, E and beta-carotene is thought to reduce cell damage and the growth of tumors in your body by interfering with the body's metabolic reactions. You could take vitamin supplements that include these, or just increase foods containing these vitamins.

Vitamin C: Oranges, black currants and other fruits, peppers, potatoes and green vegetables.

Vitamin E: Eggs, butter, seeds, nuts and oily fish.

Beta-carotene: Spinach, carrots, tomatoes and peaches.

The High-Fiber Diet

A high-fiber diet is believed to reduce the levels of estrogen in your body because it prevents excreted estrogen from being reabsorbed in the bowel. (This kind of diet is also good for constipation and bowel problems.) However, a very high-fiber diet can interfere with the absorption of nutrients and can worsen irritable bowel syndrome.

You could increase your fiber intake by eating more of the following:

- Wholegrain bread (it contains twice as much fiber as white bread)
- Fruit—a soluble fiber that inhibits the effects of cholesterol
- Vegetables such as peas, beans, lentils, leaf and root vegetables, and salads
- Unprocessed breakfast cereals made with wholewheat or grains, as well as wholewheat pasta, brown rice, oats and rye bread

The Macrobiotic Diet

Macrobiotic diets are based on eating whole, unrefined foods, such as bread, cereals, grains, pasta, vegetables, fruits, seeds, beans, certain fish and seafoods including seaweed. No refined sugar, dairy products or meat (butter, white sugar, eggs, ham and beef are thought to be particularly bad) are included. A macrobiotic diet is all about getting back to basics, that is, to *natural,* organic food lacking chemicals that might interfere with the natural processes of the body.

For more information contact the American Holistic Health Association listed in the "Useful Addresses" section at the back of book.

The Anti-Candida Diet

Candida is quite a problem for many endometriosis sufferers and can be combated by a yeast-free, sugar-free diet, designed to stop the growth of the yeastlike organism in the body called *candida albicans*.

Candida albicans lives in the urethra and alimentary canal (the passage from the mouth to the anus) of all human beings, and also in the vagina. It is similar to thrush. Your body naturally keeps *candida* in check, but when your immune system is weakened the fungus can multiply and spread.

Certain conditions—smoking too much, being overstressed, suffering from deficiencies in vitamin B_6 and C and zinc, using oral corticosteroids on a long-term basis, or taking antibiotics for long periods of time—are thought to predispose people to *candida*. Also, certain symptoms such as cravings for sweet foods, bloating and recurrent thrush are supposed to be indicative of *candida albicans*. Some researchers even believe that *candida* can get into your bloodstream, upsetting the whole body system. If the immune system is severely disrupted, very serious effects can develop that may need your urgent medical treatment.

For less serious cases you can get treatment from a nutritional or allergy specialist who may prescribe you antifungal remedies as well as certain vitamins and minerals to strengthen your immune system. You may also be put on a yeast-free diet. Treatment usually lasts one to six months, depending on how severe your case is.

Food Allergies

Allergies can make endometriosis sufferers feel even worse. Some people have found that trying out an elimination diet under the guidance of a qualified nutritional therapist can be helpful. The idea is to cut out one type of food at a time—such as wheat, dairy products and meat—to see if that relieves your symptoms, and then to gradually reintroduce the food again if it is tolerated.

Angela, who has suffered from severe endometriosis involving the bladder and the intestines, says, "As well as following a healthy diet, I try to avoid wheat and dairy products that for me result in bloating, which causes me *more* endometriosis pain. Just eating a bit of chocolate can give me a whole weekend of pain!"

Changing Your Lifestyle

The following options may also be of general help to endometriosis sufferers.

Losing Weight

If you lose excess weight you will produce less estrogen. Fat cells produce small amounts of a weaker form of estrogen. This rarely matters for younger women because their normal estrogen levels are much greater than the small amounts found in fat. However, this cellular estrogen does become important at or near menopause.

TIPS ON LOSING WEIGHT

There are any number of books and articles on sensible dieting (many of them of little worth, or just trendy). If you think there may be emotional reasons why you find it difficult to lose weight, you could try contacting a nutritionist or get a referral from your physician. You could also check with the National Eating Disorders Association (NEDA), 6655 South Yale Avenue, Tulsa, OK 74136; 918-481-4044.

Stopping Smoking

Smoking depletes the levels of vitamin B_6, as well as other B vitamins and vitamin C in the body. These vitamins are needed to counteract many of the symptoms of PMS. Women taking hormone replacement therapy will also get less benefit from it if they smoke, and will therefore get less protection against osteoporosis.

If you want to give up smoking, talk to your physician or contact the American Cancer Society (800-227-2345) or the American Lung Association (800-586-4872).

Cutting Down on Alcohol

Alcohol—whether in liquor, wine or beer—contains high levels of sugar and can contribute to mood swings. It also acts as a depressant on the nervous system, which doesn't help when fighting endometriosis.

Some sufferers develop alcohol problems, finding it the only way to blot out the pain. For confidential help, contact your local Alcoholics Anonymous organization (listed in the phone book).

Stress

Factors that cause stress contribute to endometriosis. Not only is it harder to fight an illness if you are under severe stress, but stress can also depress the immune system and recall that endometriosis is thought to be caused in part by a deficiency in the immune system. And the more stressed you are, it is believed, the more sharply you experience pain.

TIPS ON STRESS MANAGEMENT

1. Write down lists of what you need to do each day, and prioritize the tasks.

2. Don't do something just because it's expected of you —learn to say no (if you work in the business world, learn to delegate).

3. If you have a problem, talk about it. If you can't talk to a friend or relative, try counseling.

4. Give yourself breaks throughout the day to do something you enjoy, such as walking, reading or taking a relaxing bath.

5. Try to hang on to your sense of humor as much as possible. Laughter truly is often the best medicine.

6. Avoid making too many life changes at once.

7. Try not to brood over situations that you have no control over—and try not to hang on to the past.

8. Cultivate a social life.

9. Exercise regularly to reduce tension.

10. Learn to relax. You may want to learn a regular relaxation technique such as breathing exercises, yoga or massage (see Chapter 7).

11. Ask your doctor or HMO about stress management courses (see Chapter 7).

Exercise

Exercising is good for you: it keeps your body healthy and improves your circulation. Not only that, vigorous exercise (that is, exercise that gets you hot and sweaty) produces endorphins, your body's natural painkillers that make you feel more relaxed and happy.

More specifically, exercise has also been shown to help with menopausal symptoms such as mood swings, osteoporosis, constipation and other symptoms that might be shared by endometriosis sufferers. Exercise helps to keep any adhesions flexible, and might play a role in keeping your hormonal levels normal. It's also been shown to counteract many of the side effects of danazol or other drugs that you may be taking for other problems.

> Angela, who suffers severe endometriosis, says, "I try to swim two or three times a week. If I miss a session I really notice it."

> Jacqueline notes, "I felt much better when I did two or three exercise classes a week. I think that, as well as making me more relaxed and better able to fight the pain, the exercise made me feel more positive. When one class concluded and I stopped going, my pain definitely got worse."

Tranquilizers

Pills such as tranquilizers, sleeping pills and antidepressants are often prescribed for chronic pain. But they should only be used in the short term, because prolonged use of certain drugs (such as the benzodiazepines like Valium) can be addictive. They can also sometimes make the pain worse, interfere with your sleep patterns or contribute to depression. If you have a problem with addiction, you can ask for advice from your doctor or HMO on how to withdraw from your drugs slowly, or get a copy of *Free Yourself from Tranquilizers and Sleeping Pills* by Shirley Trickett (Ulysses Press). Or you could contact one of the groups listed in the "Useful Addresses" section at the back of the book.

CHAPTER SEVEN

Complementary Therapies

Complementary (or "alternative") treatments more often than not aim at treating the *whole person* rather than a disease. For this reason, such therapy is often called "holistic." When you walk into the treatment rooms of complementary therapists, they don't see you as an endometriosis sufferer. For them, endometriosis is merely the name given for the collection of symptoms you may be experiencing, but it doesn't or shouldn't define who you *are*. Complementary therapists are interested in knowing about you as a whole person: what problems you may be having (in addition to the endometriosis); what your family and lifestyle are like; what you do for a living; what other health problems you've experienced and how you dealt with them; and how you're feeling and looking right now.

Complementary therapists view illness as *dis-ease,* that is, they believe that illness comes about because of a lack of comfort or an imbalance in your life. Many nontraditional therapists believe that disease is expressed through energy blockages in the body that result in illness, and their focus is on trying to unblock that energy.

This seems a good way to approach endometriosis, particularly if the condition is in some way related to a faulty immune system (see Chapter 3). Also, as I noted earlier, endometriosis tends to set up a vicious circle of pain, tension and depression, which leads to more pain. Having a complementary therapy treatment is a good way of breaking this circle and starting a reverse process of relaxation. This leads you to feeling less tension and, in turn, less pain. If it accomplishes only this much, it is worth a try—and the chances are it will do more, since feeling better can help to strengthen your immune system, making you better able to fight endometriosis.

Some complementary therapists also say that their treatment can help balance out the hormones that are responsible for stimulating the patches of endometriosis.

There have been no scientific studies done to compare how successful complementary therapies are when compared with conventional methods. But, since endometriosis does not usually get worse over time, and in some cases it spontaneously resolves itself, it might therefore be advantageous to first give your body's own natural healing mechanisms a kick-start, before trying more invasive treatments such as surgery or drug treatments. Some people, especially those with very mild endometriosis, might prefer to start with the alternative methods before progressing to conventional treatments. Another positive thing about trying natural or holistic approaches to healing is that they are usually free from unpleasant side effects, such as those that occur with drug treatment and surgery. And natural therapies are usually less expensive than medical consultations, tests and surgery. The riskiest thing that can happen pursuing them is that your endometriosis could worsen and you could lose a little time. Bearing this in mind, it might be wise for those of you who have severe endometriosis to consult your physician before following a strict complementary approach. However, you might find that your physician is happy for you to use complementary therapies alongside conventional treatment.

For some people, just getting the one-to-one attention offered by complementary therapists—which unfortunately most traditional doctors are unable to give—can be extremely therapeutic. Whichever treatment is best for you depends on your individual situation and symptoms. What follows is a list, in alphabetical order, of some complementary therapies that have helped other endometriosis sufferers.

Acupuncture

This ancient Chinese therapy is based on the theory that our health is governed by *chi*, a flow of energy that travels in the body from one organ to another. A blockage or imbalance in this flow is thought to bring about ill health.

After taking a detailed history from you, including information about your emotional and physiological state, the acupuncturist attempts to bring about balance in the body by inserting needles into your body at specific points. These points lie along invisible energy points called meridians, which are believed to be linked to the internal organs.

Endometriosis is usually diagnosed as a "blood stagnation" condition, so the acupuncturist tries to get the blood and energy flow moving again by using the spleen meridians and liver points, all of which are found in the legs, feet and toes.

Some researchers believe that one of the ways that acupuncture works is by releasing *endorphins*, natural painkillers produced by the body, which create a local anesthesia. (If you are fearful of needles, don't worry! The needles used for acupuncture are much finer than those used for injections, they're sterile, and you generally feel only a light prick as the needle is inserted.)

Acupuncture has been known to help a number of gynecological problems, including painful periods, menopausal symptoms and PMS. There have been mixed reports from endometriosis sufferers as to its effectiveness, however. Some women have found it beneficial, whereas others said that it made their symptoms worse. Some people believe that the traditional method of acupuncture, using needles, may be more helpful than modern techniques that use electronic instruments.

For more information on acupuncture, contact the American Foundation of Traditional Chinese Medicine, 505 Beach Street, San Francisco, CA 94133; 415-776-0502.

Aromatherapy

In this form of complementary therapy, essential oils, extracted from plants for healing purposes, are used to relieve symptoms. Some essential oils have been found to have antiviral, antifungal or antibacterial properties. A vast number of different oils are used in the therapies and are taken by mouth, added to bath water, inhaled or used in massage oils. Although essential oils can be bought over the counter, it is advisable to consult a trained therapist before using them. Overdosing on certain oils, or misusing them, can be dangerous.

Your first visit to an aromatherapist usually starts with a discussion about your general health and lifestyle, including diet, exercise, posture and eating habits. You will not be diagnosed at this stage, but the therapist may test your foot reflexes as part of establishing a general picture of your health. She then chooses the appropriate oils, and then mixes and administers them through an aromatherapy massage.

Massage treatment is thought to be a particularly advantageous way for the body to absorb the oils. In this way they can reach the bloodstream more effectively. (For those in doubt, consider how traditional medicine employs this method with the use of skin patches as an effective route to get drugs into the blood stream.)

Because our sense of smell is linked directly to our brains, a scent can also have an immediate effect on our mood or muscles without our even realizing it.

An aromatherapy treatment usually lasts from 60 to 90 minutes. Someone who suffers from endometriosis might need several treatments, including continuing use of aromatherapy oils at home.

In Great Britain, where aromatherapy is much more accepted, a trial to find out how effective aromatherapy was in the treatment of endometriosis had very good results. The participants said they had an increase in pain-free days of 59 percent. The oils that the aromatherapists found particularly effective were bergamot, clary sage, cypress, fennel and geranium. Geranium apparently is very good for painful periods, as is bergamot for depression.

For more information, contact R.O.S.A. (Resource Organization for Scent and Aromatherapy), 219 Carl Street, San Francisco, CA 94117; 415-564-6785 or the American Alliance of Aromatherapy, P.O. Box 309, Depoe Bay, OR 97341; 503-392-4006 or 800-809-9850.

Bach Flower Remedies

These remedies are simple essences of particular flowers that are thought to transform negative emotions, exhibited by physical illness, into positive emotions such as optimism and joy. The principle behind the treatment is that every disorder—whether physical or psychological—arises from an inner imbalance for which nature has provided a cure in the form of healing plants, sunlight, spring water and fresh air.

Bach practitioners begin by looking at the emotional side of your illness. Because they believe that endometriosis sufferers often have suppressed anger (about something that has happened in their past or because of the way they have been treated, perhaps by the medical profession), they might treat you with gentian, which is good for suppressed anger. You may also be treated for the related stress and tension caused by the endometriosis, using the best-known application, Bach Rescue Remedy, which is taken orally or applied as cream to the painful areas such as the abdomen. Other remedies include crab apple, a cleansing remedy prescribed if a woman feels bad or guilty about having periods, or pine if there are feelings associated with having a period.

Dr. Nelson Bach, the originator, intended his remedies to be simple enough to use without consulting a professional flower therapist. You can buy them from most health food stores or herbal medicine shops. There are 38 different remedies used in all. If you are choosing a remedy for yourself, you need to examine, as honestly as possible, your mental and emotional state, your habits, attitudes and typical ways of behaving and then select the remedy most suited to you. You would normally use fewer than five remedies at a time.

For more information, contact Bach Flower Essences Educational Program, Nelson Bach, P.O. Box 0185, Baldwin, NY 11510; 800-334-0843.

Biochemical Tissue Salts

This therapy is based on the theory that the body contains 12 essential mineral salts, and if they are out of balance illness results. The mineral salts that are found lacking are then taken in minuscule forms to restore the balance. The 12 tissue salts are also listed in the homeopathic range of medicines and are prepared in the same way, although the two methods have quite different approaches. In homeopathic medicine, the remedies are prescribed to induce the symptoms of the disease, whereas with biochemical tissue salts, the salts are prescribed to make up for the mineral deficiency.

You can buy the tissue salts at health food stores (follow the dosage guidelines printed on the container). The usual method is to dissolve them on your tongue without eating, drinking or cleaning your teeth for an hour afterward. The frequency and regularity of doses is considered most important—every half hour if the symptoms are sudden and short-lived, or every two hours if they are long lasting. The tablets are absorbed quickly into the bloodstream and are said to give prompt relief to sudden illness. However, response to long-standing ailments such as endometriosis can be slow, taking six months or more.

The following tissue salts are specifically recommended for problems associated with endometriosis:

> *Kali Phos:* PMS, depression, heavy periods
>
> *Silica:* Heavy periods
>
> *Nat Mur:* Fluid retention
>
> *Nat Sulph:* Fluid retention
>
> *Mag Phos:* Painful periods
>
> *Combination S tissue salts:* Menstrual nausea

Chiropractic

Like osteopathy (see below), chiropractic involves manipulating and adjusting the spine and other joints in the body. The theory behind chiropractic medicine is that disease results from the abnormal function of the nervous system caused by misalignment of the spine and other body structures. It is often used to treat back pain and can be good for menstrual, bladder and constipation problems.

At the first consultation, a chiropractor will want to know about your medical history, as well as the endometriosis. She then examines you, feeling for areas of muscle spasm, pain and tenderness particularly in the abdominal cavity, and tries to ascertain which of your joints are moving correctly and which are not. An X-ray may then be taken to determine the position of the spine. Then she decides whether chiropractic treatment will help.

Treatment usually begins at the second visit, after the full diagnosis has been made. You are asked to undress to your underwear and to put on a robe. You then stand, sit or lie on a chiropractic table designed for manipulative therapy; various manual techniques are used such as rotation, manipulation or simple pressure application. Some patients feel relief from pain immediately, while others may experience aching soreness for a day or two before they gain relief.

The main way endometriosis sufferers benefit from chiropractic is from pain relief. A chiropractor usually concentrates on working the lumbar spine (the part of the spine located in the loin area) and the outflow to the uterus. They can manipulate areas relating to the nerve supply; for painful periods they might adjust the lumbar spine to give it more mobility. Anecdotally, chiropractors have found that nine out of ten women with endometriosis don't have a lot of movement in the lumbar spine because the pain they suffer from that condition causes muscles spasms that make the spine lock up. Your treatment might also include adjustment to the cervical spine (spine in the neck area) and the thoracic spine (spine in the chest area), both of which could have a beneficial effect on the immune system. Initially, six treatments would probably be needed for someone with endometriosis, with perhaps three of these in the first week to get things moving and loosened up.

For more information, contact the American Chiropractic Association, 1701 Clarendon Boulevard, Arlington, VA 22209; 800-986-4636.

"Healings"

No one quite knows how healing works, but with this technique a force is thought to pass through the healer's hands into the body of the patient, which helps to heal both physical and emotional problems. There are different types of healings, such as faith, spiritual and psychic healing.

Some medical experts dismiss the work of healers, pronouncing that unexplained cures are due to spontaneous remission in which the body heals itself. But for those who believe in the power of healing, it is generally thought of as a two-way process. The first thing a healer does is talk soothingly to you to induce relaxation and open your mind to the possibility of getting well again. Once a mutual bond has been established, the healer focuses her mind on her own powers, allowing them to flow freely from her to you. She may also instruct you to visualize projections of white or colored light to aid the healing process.

During the healing session, which usually takes place once a week until you improve, you usually find yourself becoming less tense and nervous. During the session you may experience feelings of heat, cold and tingling (like small electric shocks), especially on the skin over the site of the abdomen. This is taken as a sign that a healing energy is being transferred. Some patients begin to feel better as soon as the healing begins, while others may only feel benefits days later. If you want to see a healer, it is a good idea to visit one who is recommended by someone you know and trust—most do not charge a fee (being unlicensed), although a small donation may be requested.

You can get a directory of practitioners from The Universal Holistic Healers Association, P.O. Box 2022, Mount Pleasant, SC 29465; 803-849-1529.

Herbalism

Every culture throughout history has used herbs as medicine. Chinese, East Indians and American Indians all have well-developed forms of herbal medicine. Indeed, many of our own conventional medicines—from aspirin to the very latest drugs on the market—are derived from herbs, in some form or fashion.

The first consultation with an herbal therapist is usually a thorough one, encompassing your lifestyle and medical history as well as routine blood pressure and urine tests. Treatment is then prescribed in the form of syrups, tinctures (the alcoholic extract of a drug derived from a plant) or dried herbs made up into an infusion of tea. Poultices, ointments and lotions may also be used externally. An initial consultation generally lasts an hour, later appointments about half an hour.

As a rule, herbal medicines work more slowly than conventional drugs, because they are less concentrated. But as the herbs begin to enhance the body's natural healing powers, you should begin to feel better. Someone with endometriosis initially might be prescribed tinctures or infusions for three weeks, after which the treatment would be reviewed. Then, depending on how she responded, she might continue with the treatment for another month.

Some common prescriptions include false unicorn root to regulate the hormonal function, ginger or prickly ash bark to improve circulation to the pelvis, burdock or dandelion root to cleanse the system, cleavers to influence the lymphatic system, and vervain or skullcap to influence the nervous system. An adult dose is usually 5 to 10 ml. three times a day. Depending on his training, the therapist may also give dietary advice and suggest dietary supplements. For pain and discomfort, massage oils containing chamomile, which acts as an antispasmodic, might also be suggested.

Simple self-help remedies are available from health food stores or pharmacies. But for anything serious you should consult a qualified herbalist who is trained to know exactly which herb to use, how to prepare and apply it, and how much you should take.

Endometriosis sufferers have found the following self-help herbal preparations useful:

For menstrual pain and other twinges throughout the cycle: Take one pinch of powdered ginger, or a few shreds of fresh root ginger infused in a cup of boiling water, and sip the brew at regular intervals. Honey can be used to sweeten the taste. Ginger works by relieving spasms and improving circulation. Pineapple juice can also help: drink as much as you like during your period.

For bladder pain (when no infection is present): Meadowsweet tea, which is brewed just like ordinary tea, is helpful. Drink one cupful (no milk) four times a day or as required. A fresh batch should be made daily, although it can be reheated or kept in a thermos throughout the day.

For balancing hormones: Vitex agnus castus is recommended, but is best used under the supervision of an herbalist. It is thought to affect the hormones produced by the pituitary gland, and is often recommended for menstrual problems as well as infertility. It should *not* be taken at the same time as hormone treatments.

Stomach problems: Ginger (see above) taken as an infusion is good for gas and colic pains. Slippery elm tablets can also be chewed (two before each meal) to counteract the irritant effects of some drugs on the stomach.

For more information, contact the American Botanical Council, P.O. Box 201660, Austin, TX 78720; 512-331-8868 or The Herb Research Foundation, 1007 Pearl Street, Suite 200, Boulder, CO 80302; 303-449-2265 or 800-748-2617.

Chinese Herbal Remedies

Because Chinese medicine regards each person as unique, Chinese herbal medicine requires an individual diagnosis. The herbalist listens, hears, touches and sees each of her clients, and only then makes a diagnosis and comes up with a prescription.

Common diagnoses for women with endometriosis are *blood deficiency*, *blood stagnation*, a lack of *yang* (the opposite of *yin*—see ancient Chinese philosophy below), and perhaps *cold in the uterus*. A combination of herbs and acupuncture, diet, exercise and massage might be prescribed. The prescription could include *phytohormones*, which are hormones found in a gentle, plant form. Some are already used in the manufacture of hormone replacement therapy (HRT). The quantity would depend on the ratio in which these hormones were thought to be deficient.

Take Note: Ancient Chinese philosophy is based on the belief that there are two opposing but complementary forces. *Yin* is the more passive, conserving force and *yang* the more positive, thrusting force. All understanding and explanation of the world, including medical science, was based in terms of yin and yang.

Dong quai: This helps with relaxation and the pain and inflammation caused by PMS, pregnancy and menopause. It has been used for thousands of years in China to nourish and strengthen the blood and regulate periods, and is thought to be particularly good at relieving menstrual cramps.

White peony: In China, this is often used in combination with dong quai as a tonic for the nervous system. It also has a relaxing effect on the uterine muscles.

Leonuri: This herb is thought to invigorate the blood and help regulate periods. Helpful for irregular periods, premenstrual abdominal pain, infertility and water retention.

Black cohosh: An herb used by American Indians, it is used to relieve painful or delayed menstruation, ovulation pain or menstrual cramps. It is also thought to help balance female hormones.

Mexican Yam

This is a plant extract that contains diosgenin, the raw material from which progesterone can be made in a laboratory. It is thought to aid hormone balance and to reduce stress, tiredness and menopausal symptoms.

Homeopathy

This form of natural therapy—like the process used to make vaccines as well as antidotes to snake venom—is based on the idea that "like cures like." A homeopathic practitioner gives you minute amounts of whatever substance she thinks is causing your problem. This is thought to stimulate your immune system into fighting the disease.

When taking homeopathic treatments, you should avoid too much coffee and strongly flavored mints since they can interfere with the remedy's effect. Homeopaths can also offer natural remedies for the treatment of PMS and natural alternatives to hormone replacement therapy. Remedies can be taken alongside conventional drug treatments, although you must inform the homeopath of any other drugs you are taking since this could interfere with the treatment.

Most patients are treated in the same way. First you are asked to fill in a detailed questionnaire about your lifestyle, including your emotional state. You then are prescribed a homeopathic remedy, depending on the provoking situation, what sort of pain you are experiencing and where you are feeling it. Remedies are made from natural substances such as minerals, herbs, salt and even diseased tissues—all in microscopic dilutions. There are over 400 different remedies for abdominal pain alone, but common ones include *thuja* and *sepia*. Treatment takes anywhere from three months to a year.

For more information, contact the National Center for Homeopathy, 801 North Fairfax Street, Suite 306, Alexandria, VA 22314; 703-548-7790.

Meditation

There are several techniques of meditation, but all lead to the "state of meditation," a way of *being* rather than *doing*. Meditation focuses on your ability to heal yourself, to achieve clarity and peace through controlling your thoughts and calming your body.

Meditation allows you to be more conscious of your own body, to listen to what it is telling you. When meditating you enter a trance-like state, which with practice lowers your pulse and blood pressure. It can also reduce muscular tension and improve your circulation.

There are a number of private teachers or centers that can instruct you on the art of meditating. Classes are even offered by some HMOs or clinics. There are also a number of good books around to teach you the basics of concentrating on your breathing and stilling your mind. (See *Discover Meditation*, by Doriel Hall, Ulysses Press, for a basic introduction to meditation.)

TEN TIPS ON MEDITATION

1. Don't eat or drink for at least one half-hour before meditating.

2. Choose a quiet room or area where you won't be interrupted.

3. You may want to start by putting on a soothing tape and placing an object such as a favorite ornament or a photograph of a tranquil place several feet in front of you to focus on.

4. Sit comfortably but upright with your eyes open and your hands resting in your lap. This way you can relax but remain alert and controlled.

5. Concentrate on your breathing, making your diaphragm move down and your abdomen (not your chest) swell out as your breathe. Feel the air enter your nostrils and move down to fill your lungs completely; then slowly expel all the air.

6. Count as you breathe in and out, taking as long to expel the air as you did to draw it in.

7. Try to stop troublesome or stimulating thoughts from entering your mind. This is best done by filling your mind with one neutral, calming or pleasing thought or image.

8. If thoughts keep intruding, don't follow them. Merely acknowledge they have come and then resume concentration on your chosen focus.

9. Meditate for at least ten minutes. Don't worry if you find it difficult to start; with practice you will find it easier to still your mind.

10. When you have finished meditating, wiggle your feet and hands a bit before standing up, otherwise you may feel lightheaded from lowered blood pressure.

(With practice you should be able to meditate anywhere—between household chores or even on the subway to work.)

> Maria says, "I've been going to meditation at my local Buddhist center for over a year and have found that it has helped me reduce stress generally. It helps me to take my everyday life at a much slower pace. It also helps with pain relief during my period. If I wake up in the night in pain, I concentrate on my breathing and before long I've drifted off to sleep without even a painkiller!"

Osteopathy

This practice promotes health care by correcting mechanical imbalances within and between the structures of the body. (Structures in this sense refer to the muscles, bones, ligaments, organs and fascia.) This is done by restoring, maintaining and improving the working of the nervous and musculoskeletal systems. Osteopaths believe that a misalignment of bones in the spine affects the nerves and blood flow to other areas of the body, which if not corrected can cause disease. Treatment involves correcting these defects by utilizing stretching, massage and special exercises designed to relax the muscles and ligaments.

When you first visit an osteopath, he will want to know how your symptoms began and what makes them better or worse. Your medical history and any current treatment is also noted. The doctor then carries out a detailed physical examination. He observes you standing, sitting, lying down and performing certain movements such as bending forward and backward. The range and quality of the movements in the joints are assessed, and he also examines, by touch, the soft tissue, muscles and ligaments to see if they are abnormally tense or stretched. During this survey the osteopath is able to diagnose any abnormalities in the body's framework.

A treatment session usually lasts about 30 minutes, and most people find it relaxing and enjoyable. Several techniques may be used, including massaging the soft tissue to relax taut muscles and improve circulation. Exercise, advice on posture and relaxation techniques are often recommended for implementing at home between treatment sessions.

Women with endometriosis who visit an osteopath are often seeking pain relief or help with fertility problems. First they are asked about the patterns of pain and symptoms they have had. Then the abdomen and pelvic area are examined to see how much elasticity there is. Endometriosis sufferers often have abdomens that appear bound in the middle, although in fact the tension comes from the surrounding joints and ligaments. There may also be a lot of scar tissue on the peritoneum, which limits tissue movement and can cause swellings and obstructions to the blood flow. The osteopath would try to gently mobilize the tissues, to get the area to ease up as much as possible. This would also help improve the circulation in this area, as well as the lymphatic drainage and drainage from the veins. He may also externally manipulate the pelvic joints in the lower back. Some osteopaths with special training in visceral osteopathy can internally manipulate the uterus and fallopian tubes through the vagina, which may help with infertility problems. A minimum of four to six treatments are advised, especially since you won't know how successful the treatment has been until you have gone through a couple of menstrual cycles.

For more information, contact the American Osteopathic Association, 142 East Ontario Street, Chicago, IL 60611; 312-280-5800. For a basic introduction to osteopathy, read *Discover Osteopathy*, by Peta Sneddon and Paolo Coseschi (Ulysses Press).

Reflexology

This form of therapy is a health system based on the meridian theory, similar to acupuncture. It is used to relax and break down congestions, to induce circulation and energy flow and to enhance the body systems through stimulation. Reflexologists believe that the entire body is represented by points on the feet. These points are massaged or pressure is applied that stimulates a reflex action in the corresponding organ or tissue. Reflexology is particularly helpful for menstrual problems, menopause, headaches and high blood pressure.

At your first visit you are asked for a full medical history. You then lie comfortably in a reclining chair with your feet raised. Shoes and socks are removed and your feet are quickly examined for corns and calluses, which can interfere with the blood supply, or infection which could indicate disease or poor nutrition. Before starting treatment the therapist gently massages talcum into your feet to get you used to the feel of the treatment. Whatever the problem, *all* the reflex areas on both feet are massaged. Using the thumb to apply pressure, the reflexologist examines the soles, sides and tops of the feet, feeling for any special areas of tenderness that need special attention.

When a woman suffers from endometriosis, the therapist specifically looks at points relating to the uterus, fallopian tubes, ovaries, the pelvic area, the pituitary gland (which controls our hormones) and the reproductive glands (if there is a problem with infertility). By massaging these areas, she tries to restore a balance to the hormonal system and also tries to induce relaxation. Initially an endometriosis sufferer needs three or four sessions of reflexology, but in more problematic cases, six to eight treatments are preferable. Some women like to come back regularly if they find it helps with painful periods. They learn when is the best time in their cycle to return—perhaps a week before their period is due—and they keep an ongoing schedule.

For more information, contact the International Institute of Reflexology, P.O. Box 12642, St. Petersburg, FL 33733; 813-343-4811. For a basic overview, read *Discover Reflexology,* by Rosalind Oxenford (Ulysses Press).

Shiatsu

This therapy is also based on the same principles as acupuncture, but instead of using needles the practitioner massages areas where the energy flow is blocked. He may use anything from finger-and-thumb to elbow-and-knee pressure. This type of massage releases toxins and deep-seated tensions from the muscles, as well as stimulates the hormone system.

A session sometimes begins with stretching, turning and stimulating exercises to get the energy flowing. (You may also be advised to practice these exercises at home between sessions.) The therapist then applies pressure to certain points that may penetrate quite deeply but that usually feel pleasant (although sometimes they cause pain). (Pain is thought to be good because it signals an energy blockage.) The duration of the pressure, which is applied as you breathe out (because this is when your body is the most relaxed), is determined by the energy flow response. It is primarily applied by the thumb pads (not tips), since this is the most sensitive part of the hand and the easiest to control. Control is further increased by the therapist's bracing the rest of his hand lightly on your body. You may be asked to sit, or lie face down, or up, or on your side as the various points are treated. As the energy flow changes, you may feel elated or depressed for a time. Treatment may be given once a week to start with and then given at longer intervals to maintain the correct energy balance.

Shiatsu practitioners consider endometriosis a "blood stagnation" condition, particularly if pain is experienced during intercourse. There are various reasons why the blood might be stagnant: an accumulation of heat and cold congestion, or a blood or energy deficiency. If you are affected by cold congestion, this could be due to going out in cold weather poorly dressed. In cold times, you should keep your back and abdomen warmly wrapped up as well as your ankles; these areas are thought to relate to the ovaries. Blood deficiency could be a result of anemia or your having lost a lot of blood during your menstrual period. For signs of energy deficiency, the therapist looks for general lethargy, low energy and lack of vitality. To counter this, the practitioner tries to stimulate the liver and spleen meridians in your legs as well as suggests visualization techniques (like the one listed below) to release the stagnation. Women with endometriosis are also advised to avoid penetrative sex during their periods because it is believed that this could push some of the blood backward.

Self-help suggestions include a daily body scrub that stimulates the circulation and movement of blood, and avoiding stimulants such a coffee, cigarettes, sugar and chemicalized foods that do not allow your energy system to repair itself. However, with endometriosis it is advisable to consult a practitioner rather than simply employing these self-help methods.

To find a practitioner, contact The American Oriental Bodywork Therapy Association, Laurel Oak Corporate Center, 1010 Haddenfield–Berlin Road, Suite 408, Voorhees, NJ 08043; 609-782-1616.

You might also read *Shiatsu for Women*, by Ray Ridolfi and Susanne Franzen (Thorsons). For a basic overview, read *Discover Shiatsu*, by Catherine Sutton (Ulysses Press).

Stress Management

Stress is not in itself bad. In fact, life would hardly be worth living without *some* pressure and excitement. But stress becomes damaging when you can no longer handle it, when the pressure feels too much, making you feel defeated. Feeling fearful or angry over an extended period of time (which often happens with endometriosis) while suppressing the feelings only traps them in your body; they then manifest themselves in illness. Research has shown that simply dealing with the daily hassles of life, such as losing your keys or getting stuck in traffic, often lowers the body's defenses and leads to a higher risk of infection. When you are stressed, you also tend to feel pain more, which is the last thing an endometriosis sufferer wants.

Keeping stress in check often means making lifestyle changes that allow you to slow down, to distribute your load more effectively. It often means learning to relax by breathing properly, perhaps by practicing yoga or meditation. It often means learning to face up to and dealing with emotional difficulties and needs. It often means getting sufficient support for yourself. Some hospitals, HMOs and community mental health centers run courses on how to cope with stress.

> Eleanor attended a stress-management course, and reports: "I learned deep-breathing exercises and was given some relaxation tapes. I knew a lot of these techniques already because I'm a nurse, but they still helped me to put them into practice. If you can just put a chink in the vicious circle of feeling pain, fatigue, depression and then more pain, you can begin to reverse the effect."

Visualization

The therapy of visualization has been found to help cancer patients and is considered a positive technique for endometriosis sufferers as well. It involves training your mind to think of positive pictures about your body.

A number of theories have been suggested to explain how visualization works. Most are based on the premise that there is a close link between our emotions and images as well as sensations. Because emotions are accompanied by such physical sensations as deep sighs and a long face when you're unhappy, or a cry of joy accompanied by a huge smile when you're feeling exalted, visualizations can call up emotions. By altering the images through visualization, it is believed you can positively affect your feelings and physical sensations, which can lead to healing.

The British National Endometriosis Society (NES) offers a step-by-step visualization exercise to help endometriosis:

1. Begin by breathing down into your stomach and relaxing each part of your body in turn, from your toes to your head.

2. Then visualize yourself in pleasant surroundings.

3. Now visualize the weak, confused endometriosis cells lost in the wrong place, and the strong purposeful army of white cells—your body's natural defense mechanism—flooding in with increased blood flow. Picture the white cells destroying the endometriosis cells, getting rid of them, and soothing the pain while tidying up the scar tissue.

4. Next visualize your internal organs, pink and healthy, freely mobile. Visualize your hormones in balance. See yourself well and full of energy and able to achieve your goals.

This process takes about 15 minutes; it is recommended that you do it three times a day. It can also be modified to deal with other things you are feeling, such as relationship problems or pain. The idea behind the technique is that it helps you develop a positive belief system and enables you to set positive goals to alleviate your health problems.

Elizabeth, an endometriosis sufferer who benefited from acupuncture, also recommends the following books which include visualization exercises that she found helpful: *Love, Medicine and Miracles*, by Bernie Siegel; and *Guided Meditations, Explorations and Healing*, by Stephen Levine.

> Elizabeth adds: "I found that some of the meditations, such as on how to soften the pain, moved me to tears. It was also a relief to see that someone else had also tread the path I was traveling on. I also found the techniques useful in working with the pain, instead of just taking painkillers."

Yoga

This is an Asian discipline used to promote control of the mind and body. It involves learning particular postures, breathing techniques and relaxation exercises, and has been found to be especially helpful for endometriosis sufferers. Not only does it help to relax you, you can also use it to alter hormone production and restore the nervous system to good health.

Breathing is an important part of yoga; according to yoga philosophy, breath embodies the individual's *prana* or life force. Although breathing is an unconscious function, it can be consciously modified, which has an effect on your well-being. Breathing also closely reflects our various emotional states; awareness and control of breathing patterns plays a part in creating mental and emotional harmony. Also, yoga can help specifically in releasing tension. Both physical and psychological tensions are often expressed in tight muscles, which may remain contracted in a state of spasm throughout the day. Consciously stretching and releasing them enables the mind to let go of worries and stresses that originally brought about the muscle spasm. Yoga exercises also develop flexibility in the spine and the muscles of the back, which can help relieve pain, since the spine encases the nerves that lead from the brain to the trunk and limbs.

Yoga postures are also good for the endocrine system (where the hormones are made), helping to balance them out. Breathing exercises can help you get through the spasms of menstrual pain; if practiced regularly, yoga exercises may even help reduce pain. The postures also contribute to developing a healthy immune system.

For more information, contact the International Association of Yoga Therapists, 20 Sunnyside Avenue, Suite A-243, Mill Valley, CA 94941; 415-868-1147.

"Complimentary Therapy Helped Me Conceive"

Rosie, a 23-year-old waitress with endometriosis, says: "As a teenager I was told I had no chance of ever getting pregnant. From the age of 14, I suffered very badly with endometriosis and often had to go to the hospital with terrible stomach pains. I'd feel ill for two weeks of every month. I eventually underwent a laparoscopy and was diagnosed with endometriosis. My physician warned me it would affect my fertility because I

How to Choose a Practitioner

Ask your physician or a friend to recommend a practitioner. Make sure they are a member of a recognized registered organization with a code of practice.

Ask if they have treated anyone with endometriosis before.

Look for someone you like and feel comfortable with.

Ask how many treatments you might expect, the approximate cost and whether they offer a sliding scale of fees.

Note: Don't expect an instant cure. Most alternative therapies are gentle and take a while to work.

had severe endometriosis on my right ovary. So I resigned myself to the fact that I'd only be a surrogate mother to other people's children. Fortunately, when I met my fiancé four years ago he was very understanding about it.

"However, after we'd been together a few years we decided to try to conceive anyway. When after a few months nothing happened, I decided to try complementary medicine, to help ease the endometriosis pain.

"Over the years I'd been on every drug under the sun for endometriosis. I even had to take the male hormone danazol for a while, which made me feel very sick. I'd had enough of the whole thing and wanted to do something more natural and positive. So I was referred to a homeopathic clinic. The good thing about it was that they wanted to know all about me, to hear my whole story, and I finally felt someone was listening. They also gave me a simple remedy called Natrum Muriaticum, which is made from sea salt, to dissolve under my tongue once a month at the beginning of my cycle. It's supposed to be a good treatment for people who hold feelings in, and I found I was soon feeling so much better. But there was still no baby.

"After that, I was anxious to continue with complementary therapy and so I went to see an acupuncturist. She used a range of points on my body including my toes and thumbs. She also wanted to know about my childhood and any problems I'd had. Talking made me feel so much more relaxed and happy.

"Just three months after starting acupuncture I found myself feeling thirsty. At first I thought nothing of it and then I decided to do a home pregnancy test. I couldn't believe it when it turned out to be positive! I was really in shock. Now I've got my hands full with six-month-old Dan. But all through the pregnancy I couldn't believe I was going to be a mother until I actually held him in my arms."

When to Consider Drugs or Surgical Treatments

If you have tried the natural approaches described in this chapter and the previous one—at least, those that seem appropriate for you—and still have not found relief from the pain of endometriosis, you may need to seek help from drug therapy or surgery. While these can be more problematical than natural treatments, they may be necessary for severe cases. Part III presents the case for such medical treatment and explains the options available to you.

PART THREE
Conventional Approaches

CHAPTER EIGHT

Drug Treatments

How Does Drug Treatment Work?

Many different types of drugs are available on the market for the treatment of endometriosis. But the main aim of all of them is to stop your periods for six to nine months. The theory behind this is that once the patches of endometriosis are no longer stimulated by hormones released before or during your period, these patches will shrink and stop causing pain. Then, when your menstrual cycle returns to normal, endometriosis is less likely to occur.

The main hormone thought to stimulate endometriosis is the female sex hormone estrogen, and thus much of the treatment is aimed at reducing the amounts of estrogen in your body. For this reason, too, many of the drugs prescribed for endometriosis aim to mimic the states of menopause or pregnancy. That's because when a woman is pregnant or menopausal she has smaller amounts of estrogen in her body, and endometrial deposits seem to regress in these states.

Which Drug Should I Take?

Obviously, the best drug to take is the one that is the most effective for you and that has the fewest side effects. Side effects vary from person to person, and the only way to find out what they are for you (if there are any) is to take the drug for a while. Physicians usually recommend that you try a drug out for six months, and you are usually asked to come in for a follow-up visit after three months to see how you are doing. Allowing for the fact that your body is likely to take a little while to adjust when it is suddenly plunged into a state of false menopause or pregnancy, it's a good idea to report any unwanted side effects to your doctor, if only to reassure yourself that they are normal.

If the side effects are severe, however, you should stop treatment *immediately*. Symptoms to watch out for include an increase in your blood pressure, tightness in your chest or changes in your voice.

The effectiveness of a drug differs from person to person. Physicians usually suggest a drug that they think is suitable based on their knowledge of endometriosis. But you don't have to agree automatically to take what your physician suggests, and you can ask for a list of the side effects before you decide. If, once you have tried a drug, you discover that it doesn't suit you, you can try others until you find the one you like best.

Warning: *If you are pregnant, you should not be taking these drugs because they can cause fetal abnormalities.*

Remember that, with any drug treatment, you may not experience side effects at all, or you may experience one or two side effects—but it is very rare to have all of them!

What Are the Advantages of Drug Treatment?

- Certain drug treatments can get rid of the pain. Such treatment has been found to successfully treat pain in 80 to 90 percent of the cases.

- Drug therapy treats microscopic patches of endometriosis.

- Drug treatment allows you to avoid the upheaval of going into the hospital for surgery and the risk of post-operative adhesions (that is, internal areas that some-times stick together following surgery, because of the local inflammation surgery may cause).

What Are the Disadvantages of Drug Treatment?

- Drug treatment doesn't always get rid of large or deeply embedded endometriosis.

- You may experience unpleasant side effects.

- The long-term effects of drug treatment are not really known.

- It can be a hassle remembering to take tablets or use nasal sprays, or undergoing uncomfortable injections.

What follows is a description of the current drugs prescribed for endometriosis, together with some of the pros and cons of each.

The Contraceptive Pill

What Is the Contraceptive Pill?

There are many different brands of the Pill on the market, some of the most common being *Loestrin*, *Norcept*, *Ortho-Novum* and *Norinyl*.

The combined contraceptive pill is often the first option suggested to an endometriosis sufferer, especially if you haven't started a family. It is the safest way to buy time, relieving the pain until you have made a decision on whether or not to have children. Obviously, many young women don't know whether they want children, so it seems wise to keep your options open as long as possible.

The combined contraceptive pill is basically made up of different combinations of estrogen and progesterone. These have the effect of mimicking pregnancy, causing a shrinking in the lining of the uterus (along with any endometrial deposits present). When used to treat endometriosis, the Pill is usually taken *continuously* for four to six months without the usual seven-day monthly break that you have when taking it for contraceptive purposes. If successful, it can be continued until a woman wishes to become pregnant or wants a "natural" break.

Who Takes the Pill?

Any woman can take the Pill, although it is often prescribed to teenagers and young women with a mild form of the disease, and sometimes to women who have recurrent ovarian cysts. If you have not had problems taking the Pill, it might be well worth considering.

Who Can't Take It?

- Women with high blood pressure

- Women who are at risk of developing blood clots

- As with normal contraceptive pills, smokers and women over 35 (who are more at risk if they take the combined contraception pill over a long period of time).

What Are the Side Effects?

Several side effects may be observed, depending on the brand you take. But the commonly reported ones are generally:

- Weight gain

- Nausea

- Breast tenderness and enlargement

- Depression

- Headaches

- Loss of sexual drive

How Successful Is It?

The Pill is not thought to be as effective in treating endometriosis as progestogens, androgens or GnRH analogues (see below). Many women find they have problems with breakthrough bleeding on the Pill, while some even say that it doesn't get rid of their pain. But it can relieve symptoms in many women and is certainly worth a try as a first option.

Androgenic Drugs (Male-Type Hormones)

What Is Danazol?

Danazol (marketed as *Danocrine*) was until recently the most common drug used for the treatment of endometriosis. A synthetic form of the male hormone testosterone, danazol works by changing your body chemistry so that it is similar to a menopausal state, with low estrogen and high androgen (male hormone) levels. It acts directly on the ovaries by interfering with the enzymes responsible for the production of the female hormones estrogen and progesterone. As mentioned before, low amounts of estrogen discourage the growth of more endometriosis and help to shrink already established patches. Danazol can also be used to treat women with breast disease, heavy periods and premenstrual syndrome.

One reasons doctors often prescribe danazol is that it is relatively inexpensive when compared to other treatments, such as progestogens and GnRH analogues (more on these later).

Who Usually Takes Danazol?

In addition to relieving pain, some women are given short courses of danazol before surgery to remove endometrial deposits thought to be causing infertility, or before undergoing a hysterectomy and removal of the ovaries. In both cases, the treatment aims to decrease the size and number of endometriosis patches, making surgery easier.

> Megan says, "I actually had drug treatment after I'd had surgery to remove fibroid and severe adhesions in my abdominal cavity. My doctor explained that it was to suppress my cycle for longer and to give my uterus the best chance of recovering

before my periods started again. I was a bit disappointed, though, when my periods returned, since they were still very painful."

Who Can't Take Danazol?

Women who:

- Are pregnant or breastfeeding
- Have the blood clotting disorder thromboembolic disease
- Have male hormone–dependent tumors
- Have heart, liver or kidney problems
- Have abnormal, undiagnosed vaginal bleeding
- Have porphyria (a rare metabolic disease)
- Have undiagnosed genital bleeding

What Dose Should I Be On?

Women with mild endometriosis are usually given between 200 and 400 mg. a day; women with moderate to severe forms take up to 800 mg. a day.

Once your symptoms begin to clear up, however, the dose may be reduced. The drug is usually started on the first day of your period, to make sure you're not pregnant. Although your periods usually stop when you take danazol, barrier contraception should also be used as a precaution because the drug can cause damage to a fetus.

What Are the Side Effects of Danazol?

Many women stop danazol because of the side effects, and three out of four women will notice at least one. The most common one reported is weight gain, with the average gain being eight pounds by women taking the higher dose.

The other most common side effects are:

- ◆ Decreased breast size
- ◆ Mild hirsutism (increased hair growth)
- ◆ Flushing
- ◆ Mood change
- ◆ Oily skin
- ◆ Depression
- ◆ Sweating
- ◆ Decreased libido

Some of the side effects, such as hot flushes and a dry vagina, are associated with being in a simulated state of menopause. Others have to do with making the body more masculine, such as increased hair and voice changes. If voice changes do occur, *notify your physician immediately* because it can be permanent. Some sufferers also report joint pain, although there's no official study on this.

Because danazol affects the blood fats and liver function, it is not a good idea to take it over a long period of time, because the medical community does not have information on its long-term effects.

One of the widely reported symptoms, although not documented, is nausea.

> Joanne, a 27-year-old customer service supervisor who was diagnosed as having an endometriosis nodule between the bowel and the uterus, says: "I tried danazol for three weeks, but it made me sick every day and there was just no way I could continue like that. So I kept switching drugs until I found one I could tolerate."

How Successful Is It?

Many women's symptoms improve within four to eight weeks after starting the treatment, and women suffering particularly from pelvic pain notice a significant improvement.

Using danazol, women with mild endometriosis who want to get pregnant also have a better chance of conceiving.

Take note! Weight gain can be reduced by starting a diet-and-exercise program *before* treatment. Many women have also found that vitamin B_6 and Evening Primrose oil can counteract some of the side effects such as tiredness, depression, water retention and mood swings (more on this in Chapter 6).

Progestins

What Are Progestins?

Progesterone is a female hormone responsible for preparing the uterus for pregnancy. In its synthetic form it can also cause the uterine lining to shrink and, along with it, any other endometrial deposits. "Progestin" is basically the name given to any substance that has the same effects as the natural hormone progesterone. Progestins trick the body into thinking it's pregnant, resulting in a lowering of the levels of estrogen in the body, which helps to relieve endometriosis. Progestin is less commonly used than danazol, but is a useful alternative —especially because the side effects tend to be less severe.

Who Can't Take It?

In addition to some of the general restrictions already mentioned for drug treatments (such as not being pregnant or breastfeeding), you should stop *immediately* if you experience any of the following:

- Migraines
- Pain or tightness of the chest
- Jaundice
- Itching
- High blood pressure
- If you are due for an operation in the next six weeks

In certain circumstances, you also shouldn't take a particular brand of progestin. If you suffer from liver problems or thrombosis, you should inform your physician. You should always check with your doctor before taking a drug to learn the contraindications (that is, symptoms or conditions that make a particular treatment inadvisable).

What Dose Should I Be On?

The most common progestin prescribed is Medroxyprogesterone Acetate (marketed as: *Depo-Provera, Amen, Cycrin, Premphase, Prempro, Provera Tablets* and *Medroxyprogesterone*).

Medroxyprogesterone Acetate is usually taken in the form of a 10 to 30 mg. tablets a day for at least three months, but for not more than six months. Studies have shown that weight gain tends to be lower than with danazol, although sufferers are likely to have more problems with fluid retention. Other side effects include:

- Depression
- Heavier periods during the first few periods
- Back pain
- Sore breasts
- Bloating, fluid retention
- Dizziness and headaches
- Cramps
- Breakthrough bleeding
- Nausea
- Lethargy

When larger doses (100 mg. or more per day) of progestin are used, it can also cause:

- Milk production from breasts
- Hair loss
- Gastric upsets
- Dry vagina

Fiona says: "I put on several pounds, and my breasts even began to produce milk! I got incredibly tired and fell asleep as soon as I got home from work. But I battled on, taking it for six months, because anything was better than horrible menstrual pains."

Ruth, a 29-year-old with endometriosis, says, "I've been on Provera for a couple of years—first in tablet form and now as an injection every 12 weeks. I've put on weight and find I get a very flaky scalp. I also suffered a little from dizziness and nausea to start with, but that seems to have settled down. Aside from that, I'm quite happy with it."

Take note: The side effects are generally mild with Medroxyprogesterone Acetate, but it must be taken with adequate medical supervision, especially because it can cause fluid-retention problems that may affect certain women, such as those with asthma, diabetes, epilepsy, renal dysfunction, depression and cardiac dysfunction.

Norethindrone

Norethindrone is sold under the brand name *Aygestin*. The dosage is a 5 mg. tablet a day, for four to six months. The dosage is usually increased gradually until bleeding and spotting stops.

The side effects include:

- Nausea and bloating
- Breakthrough bleeding
- Change in menstrual flow
- Spotting
- Changes in weight (increase and decrease)
- Rash
- Amenorrhea
- Mental depression
- Exacerbation of epilepsy and migraine

- Possible change in liver function (with higher doses)

- Possible small rise in body temperature

Megan says: "I felt awful on it. I suffered from dizziness, tiredness and found it hard to concentrate. I felt sort of spaced-out all the time, and not really like myself. I also got hot flashes and felt very depressed and anxious most of the time."

The Progestin Coil

Some women are now being treated with a coil called Mirena *(progestasert)*, which carries a progestin (38 mg. of progesterone) used in oral contraceptives and hormone replacement therapy (HRT). It works by releasing a very low daily dose of the hormone directly into the uterus. The coil itself also prevents the growth of the uterine lining and thickens the cervical mucus, which prevents the passage of sperm and suppresses ovulation in some women.

As the contraceptive pill is often the first line of treatment in the management of endometriosis, it may well be that the progestin coil could be equally effective. The manufacturer says that, although it is not specifically licensed for the treatment of endometriosis, it is an option many gynecologists are now using or considering.

Take note! Generally, progestogens seem to be as effective as danazol (sometimes slightly more so), but with fewer side effects.

GnRH Analogues

What Are GnRH Analogues?

GnRH analogues work by interfering with the action of a natural hormone called *GnRH,* which stands for *gonadotrophin-releasing hormone.* This hormone triggers the release from the pituitary gland of two other hormones—FSH (follicle-stimulating hormone) and LH (luteinizing hormone)—which in turn set the menstrual cycle in action (see Chapter 1). GnRH analogues interfere with normal hormone production, causing periods to stop, resulting in a medically induced meno-pause. Its effect is similar to that of removing the ovaries (only in *this* case it can be reversed).

Who Takes Them?

GnRH analogues are available to most women, and are becoming more popular as a treatment for endometriosis because the side effects seem to be less severe than with other drug treatments, especially the male hormone derivative.

Who Can't Take Them?

Women who are:

* Pregnant or breastfeeding
* Suffering from abnormal vaginal bleeding
* Allergic to the drug, or sensitive to other GnRH ana-logues

Also see the precautions of individual drugs listed below.

What Dose Should I Take?

Unfortunately, GnRH analogues cannot be given by mouth because they break down too quickly before having an effect. So they are usu-ally taken in the form of nasal sprays, as slow-release implants or as an intramuscular injection. But they should not be taken if you are pregnant, and barrier methods of contraception should always be con-tinued. The most common GnRH analogues are goserelin (trade name: *Zoladex*), leuprolide acetate (trade name: *Lupron Depot*) and nafarelin (trade name: *Synarel*), each of which we will now look at in turn.

Goserelin

This drug (trade name: *Zoladex*) usually comes in an injection form: 3.6 mg. are injected once a month, for a period of six months, under the skin at the front of the abdomen, using a local anesthetic. The goserelin is then gradually released into the body during the month.

Reported side effects include:

- Hot flashes
- Loss of sex drive
- Headaches
- Depression
- Sweating
- Dry vagina
- Mood changes
- Changes in breast size

Take note: Occasionally, women taking goserelin may enter menopause and never get their periods back afterward. Most women also suffer a reduction in bone density during treatment, which can be partially reversed after treatment finishes. For this reason, women with a known metabolic bone disease are advised not to take it.

> Karen, who took Zoladex for three months prior to laser surgery, says: "Once a month I was given a local anesthetic and then the Zoladex was injected into my belly, in the form of a small pellet. I felt quite tender and bruised afterward. The side effects included hot flashes, a depressive feeling and night sweats."

Leuprolide Acetate

This drug (trade name: *Lupron Depot*) is administered once a month by the injection of a 3.75 mg. dose into the arm, the abdominal wall or the thigh; injections continue for six months. It's sometimes prescribed to women 12 weeks before pelvic surgery.

The reported side effects include:

- Hot flashes

- Insomnia
- Loss of sex drive
- Nausea
- Dry vagina
- Loss of bone density
- Weight gain
- Fluid retention
- Mood changes
- Headaches

Nafarelin

This drug (trade name: *Synarel*) is usually taken in the form of two 200 mcg. sprays per day (400 mcg. in total) for six months. Trials show that it works as well as danazol, but with a lower percentage of side effects.

Side effects may include:

- Hot flashes
- Dry vagina
- Mood swings
- Reduction in breast size
- Changes in sex drive
- Headaches
- Muscle pains
- Nasal irritation

Linda says, "I only took nafarelin for two months, but stopped it because it gave me terrible headaches and made me feel very dizzy."

Angela too found it unsuitable: "It gave me mood swings and hot flashes, and I felt totally depressed on it; so I only took it for a month."

Take note: A number of the side effects of GnRH analogues are associated with menopausal symptoms, such as hot flashes, which occur in 74 to 98 percent of women. One problem with these drugs is that the symptoms often get worse for a short time before they get better.

Many doctors are also worried about the long-term effects of thinning bones and the increased risk of heart attacks due to the lack of estrogen when taking these drugs.

Normal menopausal women still have a certain amount of estrogen that can protect them against these things. For this reason, some doctors are prescribing a low dose of hormone replacement therapy to counteract the possible bone-thinning effects of these drugs.

Why Don't Some Treatments Work?

Having drug treatment alone doesn't always work. This is because the drugs may have difficulty in attacking deeply embedded endometrial deposits, especially those that have glands and the ability to produce new endometrial cells and endometriomas (endometrial cysts on the ovary). Six months of treatment may also not be enough to be effective. For this reason, some women take lower doses for longer periods, or are happy to take the risk of being on treatment for longer. If in doubt, you should speak to your physician about whether taking continuous medication with small breaks in between might be an option for you.

Painkillers for Endometriosis

What Is the Best Way to Take Painkillers?

It's a good idea to take painkillers with something that will line your stomach wall, such as a meal, or a glass of milk and a cracker. Never take them on an empty stomach unless it is indicated.

Problems with Painkillers

Often women with endometriosis don't find over-the-counter drugs very useful, especially as, over time, they seem to lose their effect.

However, it's not a good idea to take stronger prescription painkillers for an extended length of time, because they can become addictive. Many endometriosis sufferers find it's a good idea to juggle different strengths of painkillers around to suit their needs. For instance, they reserve the very strong ones only for very bad days. You should feel free to discuss with your doctor any painkillers you are taking that don't seem to be working. It might also be a good idea to investigate alternative methods of relieving pain (see Chapters 6 and 7).

What Are the Side Effects?

Most painkillers can irritate the stomach lining, causing nausea and vomiting, and in some cases lead to coughing up or passing blood. Sometimes they can also cause constipation or diarrhea.

Some of these side effects can be offset by taking a simple antinausea tablet, such as a motion-sickness pill. Alternatively, you could try senna tablets, which are a natural laxative, or lactulose, a prescription-only syrup that speeds up the action of the intestine, giving extra lubrication to the feces. Including fiber in your diet is also a good idea. As a general rule, if after trying a painkiller for two weeks it has no effect, it is unlikely that it will help you and it would be worthwhile trying a different one.

Over-the-Counter Painkillers

(NSAIDs: See under prescribed drugs below.)

Acetaminophen: This acts as a painkiller but isn't an anti-inflammatory. It is probably the easiest painkiller to take and has fewer side effects than other analgesics (a more technical term for a painkiller). However, acetaminophen may be less effective for more than mild pain.

Aspirin: Reduces inflammation and fever, but can cause stomach irritation, so should be taken with food or milk, or as a soluble tablet. It is good for mild to moderate pain.

Ibuprofen: Another popular anti-inflammatory or NSAID. It's a mild painkiller, but it can also irritate the stomach.

What Is DLPA?

DLPA is a nutritional painkiller that is a mixture of two forms of phenylalanine, an amino acid found in food proteins.

HOW DOES IT WORK?

If taken regularly, DLPA is thought to protect and strengthen our body's own natural painkillers (endorphins). Because phenylalanine is one of the eight essential amino acids that occur naturally in our bodies, DLPA isn't classified as a drug but rather as a nutritional supplement. It has been found to help with acute and chronic pain, as well as with lower back pain, premenstrual cramps and joint pains, among other things.

HOW DO YOU TAKE DLPA?

DLPA tablets are usually taken for several weeks rather than just at the time when you are experiencing pain. The dose is usually 375 mg. capsules three times a day at mealtimes. Once you start to feel the painkilling effect, you can either reduce the dose or stop taking the tablets until the next time you need them.

WHAT ARE THE ADVANTAGES OF DLPA?

- It can have an effect equal to taking morphine, but is not addictive.

- It can be used in conjunction with drugs and other therapies such as acupuncture.

- It helps with the depression that often accompanies chronic pain.

- Pain relief can continue for up to a month after stopping the treatment.

WHAT ARE THE DISADVANTAGES OF DLPA?

- It doesn't work for everyone—30 percent of users get little or no relief.

- It can cause severe indigestion.

- It shouldn't be taken if you are pregnant, if you suffer from high blood pressure or if you are on monoamineoxidase (MAO) inhibitor drugs for depression.

Leora, 29, says, "I've found I have absolutely no side effects with DLPA and I'm very happy with it. I usually take it over three weeks and find that it provides pain relief for the following three months."

Prescribed Painkillers

If over-the-counter painkillers don't work, your doctor might prescribe any of the following stronger painkillers.

Mild to moderate strength: Co-analgesics, such as Tylenol with codeine, which are a mixture of codeine and acetaminophen. Distalgesics such as coproxamol, which contain a mixture of propoxyphene hydrochloride (Darvon) and acetaminophen, are also of a similar strength.

Moderate to strong: Dihydrocodeine is a moderate to strong painkiller, but can cause constipation and dependency.

The strongest: Opiates or opiods, such as morphine and Demerol. These are prescribed only for severe pain, and are not suitable for long-term use, as you can become dependent quickly, even in low doses.

Tranquilizers, sleeping pills and antidepressants: These may also be prescribed for chronic pain. They include diazepam (Valium) and carbemazepine (Tegretol), an antianxiety drug that can control muscle spasms and that may be used for nerve pain.

NSAIDs (Nonsteroidal Anti-Inflammatory Drugs)

Brand names include *Anaprox, Anaprox DS* and *Naprosyn*. NSAIDs are a mild type of painkiller that work by inhibiting the production of prostaglandins in the body. They can be bought over-the-counter, although the stronger versions are only available by prescription.

Prostaglandins are chemicals made by body tissues; they send "messages" to the uterus, making it shrink, and causing the uterine walls to contract during periods or childbirth. They're also part of the body's natural healing mechanism, because they go to injury sites and activate the pain receptors, causing inflammation. It's thought endometriosis sufferers have *extra* prostaglandins, because these can be produced by endometriotic tissues.

The idea behind NSAIDs is that by introducing drugs that block prostaglandins you will suffer less pain. They work best, however, if they are taken early in the pain cycle. For instance, if you know you usually experience pain on Day 21 of your menstrual cycle, it's a good idea to start taking them on Day 20.

CHAPTER NINE

Surgery

Deciding on Surgery

Surgery, as you undoubtedly know, is the branch of medicine that treats disease or injury by an operation involving cutting or manipulating the infected parts. In recent years many surgical techniques and innovations have been developed to treat endometriosis—but unfortunately there are no studies on whether surgery is more effective than drug treatment. The decision whether or not to have surgery needs careful consideration and should be based on your individual situation: how bad is your endometriosis; whether you've had children already; costs and possibly time off work or away from household chores; family concerns and living conditions; and many other factors. Surgery is often used in conjunction with drug treatment, which is often given before an operation to reduce the number of endometrial deposits requiring surgery.

Surgery for endometriosis is divided into the following two categories:

* *Conservative surgery:* This is when patches of endometriotic tissue, cysts and adhesions are removed, leaving your organs intact so that it is still possible for you to become pregnant. The operations are a laparoscopy (see Chapter 4), a laparotomy, laser laparoscopy and microsurgery.

* *Definitive or radical surgery:* When your uterus, fallopian tubes and ovaries are removed. These operations are described in Chapter 10.

Why Have Surgery?

Surgery is usually advised in the following situations, when:

* Drug treatment hasn't worked

* Your symptoms have returned after drug treatment

* Reconstruction of an organ is needed as a treatment for infertility

* Your endometriosis is severe, includes adhesions and is affecting other important organs such as the bowel or intestines

* Your family is complete

* You specifically request surgery

What Are the Advantages of Surgery?

* It's the only way to remove large, deeply embedded patches of endometriosis, cysts and adhesions.

* There are no side effects, as with drugs.

* The treatment can result in immediate pain relief.

* New methods such as laser surgery are now so improved that there is a minimal risk of the damage (such as creating adhesions), which was sometimes caused during conventional surgery.

What Are the Disadvantages of Surgery?

- ◆ It requires time off work for the surgery and recovery.

- ◆ You have to undergo an anesthetic.

- ◆ The surgeon can only remove what he or she can see (so microscopic deposits of endometriosis can't be removed).

- ◆ It's sometimes difficult to recognize endometriosis.

- ◆ The endometriosis may be close to sensitive organs, such as the bowel, and can't be removed for fear of damaging the organ.

- ◆ Surgery might cause more damage—it can cause additional adhesions, which can reduce fertility.

- ◆ Endometriosis may still recur.

Laparotomy

What Is a Laparotomy?

A *laparotomy* is a major operation to open the abdomen, remove endometrial sites and correct any other problems with the reproductive organs. It's not as popular as it used to be because of the development of laparoscopy (see Chapter 4), but is still considered suitable if:

- ◆ You have experienced complications during a laparoscopy

- ◆ You suffer from severe endometriosis and adhesions

- ◆ You need more extensive work done on other organs

- ◆ You are overweight, which can make a laparoscopy difficult

What Happens During a Laparotomy?

You undergo a general anesthetic, after which a 10- to 15-centimeter cut is made below the bikini line. Any ovarian cysts or patches of endometriosis are removed, and if possible, adhesions are separated and removed. This is done by using cauterizing (heat) treatment (diathermy), incisions or laser. During the operation, a procedure called *presacral neurectomy* may also be carried out if you suffer from severely debilitating pain. This involves cutting a bundle of nonessential nerves so that some of the pain messengers from the pelvis no longer reach the brain. However, this can only be done with your consent, and its results so far have not been very successful. A presacral neurectomy is advisable *only* as a last resort.

What Are the Advantages of a Laparotomy?

- Open surgery gives the surgeon a better view of your pelvic organs.

- There is less risk of damage to other organs.

- Laser surgery can also be used during the operation.

- It alleviates pelvic pain in over 80 percent of the cases, and in women suffering from infertility, the pregnancy rate after a laparotomy is about 38 percent of women with severe endometriosis (stage III or IV).

What Are the Disadvantages of a Laparotomy?

- Because of the larger cut, there is more risk of adhesions forming afterward.

- There is a longer recovery time and a more extensive scar than with a laparoscopy.

- If extensive surgery is needed, there's more risk of infection and damage to the pelvic organs.

- Endometriosis recurs within five years in 35 percent of the women who have undergone a laparotomy.

"I Had a Laparotomy"

Megan went in for a laparoscopy, but then proceeded to a laparotomy because it was difficult to remove the dense adhesions.

She says, "I think I was in the operating room for quite a long time. I went in at 2 p.m. and didn't wake up until 8 p.m. They told me then that I'd had extensive endometriosis on my uterus and ovaries, and that this had been lasered off and the adhesions removed. But unfortunately they had to leave an adhesion that was sticking my uterus to the bowel, because they were worried about damaging the bowel.

"When I woke up I had a scar about seven inches long. I also had a small blood transfusion going into one arm because I'd lost so much blood, and an antibiotic drip in the other arm. I also had a deep stomach drain coming out of the scar, which drained debris into a bottle beneath my bed.

"I had a catheter in place too, which gave me the feeling that I was going to the bathroom all the time, but as soon I got used to it they took it out. I was in the hospital for six days, during which time I had painkilling injections every three hours.

"I was told it would take me about six weeks to recover and that I shouldn't lift anything heavy until then, so I arranged for friends to do my shopping for me. Within three weeks I was mobile again and able to walk around. It did take three weeks, though, for the pain to go away.

"All in all I'd say it took me about ten weeks to recover. Fortunately I'd arranged everything well, making sure people could come in and see me and help me with the housework. I also cleaned the house from top to bottom before going in to make it easier for me when I came out.

"I did feel a little depressed afterward, as though I'd been violated because someone had touched my insides, and I had a few flashbacks of the operation. No one tells you about that!"

Laser Laparoscopy?

What Is a Laser Laparoscopy?

The word *laser* is an acronym for "light amplification by stimulated emission of radiation." Various substances give out a very thin beam of light when they are stimulated by an electrical charge. This beam of light can then be controlled using mirrors, and very precisely directed down a laparoscope onto an area to burn away endometrial tissue or vaporize it (a type of melting). These lasers are so accurate that it is possible for them to cut grooves into a human hair. Because they are so precise, when used properly they do not cause damage to surrounding tissues during treatment.

There are four main types of laser:

- *The carbon dioxide laser:* Used for treating mild to moderate endometriosis because it is easy to control

- *The argon laser:* For vaporizing (melting) large cysts and sealing blood vessels

- *The KTP (potassium titanyl phosphate) laser:* Penetrates deeply and so is good for treating large, deeply embedded cysts that are difficult to get at

- *The nd-YAG (neodymium–yttrium aluminum garnet) laser:* Used to destroy large deposits because it penetrates deeply into tissues

What Happens During a Laser Laparoscopy?

In addition to the two cuts made during a laparoscopy (through which the laparoscope and the handling instruments are passed, as described in Chapter 4), two more tiny incisions are made on either side of the abdomen, below the bikini line. One is for the laser and the other for the venting device that allows waste gases and tissue out of the abdomen and through which fluid is passed to wash out the cavity. The laser is then used to divide adhesions, vaporize deposits of endometriosis, drain cysts and improve fertility by reconstructive surgery.

As with a laparoscopy, these incisions are closed afterward with a single stitch or staple. The procedure may also involve the division of uterine nerves with a laser, often referred to as *LUNA* (laparascopic uterine nerve ablation), which stops some of the pelvic pain messages from getting to the brain.

Jackie says, "When I had my second laser laparoscopy because of severe endometriosis, they also did a LUNA treatment to help with the pain relief, and the symptoms did improve for a while. Afterward I'd get a deep, strong aching pain around this area when walking or exercising. I also found that I experienced some pain on orgasm afterward. However, my symptoms generally did improve for a while."

What Are the Advantages of a Laser Laparoscopy?

* Laser burns heal very quickly, with minimal scar tissue and bleeding.

* There is less disruption to your life because a laser laparoscopy can usually be done during a 24- to 48-hour hospital stay.

* It has a 70 percent success rate in relieving abdominal pain.

* It can increase your chances of pregnancy, sometimes as much as 75 percent.

What Are the Disadvantages of a Laser Laparoscopy?

* New lesions can form at new sites after treatment.

* There's a small risk of damage to the bowel, bladder or blood vessels when the laparoscope is inserted or if a laser is inaccurately used, which can lead to the need for a laparotomy to correct them.

* Surgery may be no more effective than drug treatment.

"I Had a Laser Laparoscopy"

Vanessa says: "After a laparoscopy and two scans revealed that one of my ovaries was inflamed, I was admitted to the hospital for laser surgery. After being visited by just about everyone—the surgeon, the anesthetist and so on—I was given an anesthetic and taken down to the operating room. I believe I was in the operating room for about five hours.

"I woke up to find two incisions around my navel area and a third on the right-hand side of my stomach. I must admit the pain was terrible. I was told it would take two weeks to recover, but really it took me over six. My mother had to look after me for the following two weeks because I could hardly move from my bed because of the pain. She even had to wash my hair for me!

"I also had to wear a sanitary napkin because of the bleeding from the laser sites. I was relieved, though, that they had found some endometriosis, because my previous physician had been very skeptical. They found it in front of and behind my uterus, and said they had just gotten to it in time before it spread to my ovaries! I was pain free for five months, but unfortunately it then returned so I'm going to have the operation repeated."

Microsurgery

This form of surgery is a new technique still being researched that involves special Teflon-coated metal tools that don't cause abrasions and adhesions because of their nonstick surface. Incisions are made with a hot wire, which cuts as well as seals, and the "debris" is then removed by suction. The procedure is highly methodical, involving very neat stitching, which works well for separating adhesions and not replacing them with new ones. Sometimes artificial patches are used to prevent organs from sticking together again. The other advantage of this method is that there is less (slightly) risk of infection occurring afterward.

Lynne had three hours of microsurgery to separate adhesions and cauterize the endometriosis. She says, "I found it didn't hurt as much after microsurgery as with ordinary surgery. The sites also definitely healed quicker, and I wasn't in as much pain."

Operations: General Hints and Tips

What to Ask Before Any Operation

It is important to ask your physician exactly what type of operation you are undergoing, and to have anything explained that you don't understand. You might also want to find out the following:

- ◆ How long will you stay in hospital, and how long will it take to recover?

- ◆ What action will be taken if complications occur, that is, will a laparotomy then be carried out? (When signing the operation consent form, you can ask specifically that a hysterectomy and/or the removal of the ovaries *not* be performed.)

- ◆ What symptoms can you expect afterward?

- ◆ Is the surgeon fully trained in laparoscopic technique? (You might also want to ask how many laparoscopies he or she has performed.)

Take Note!

Before surgery it is important to be sure that you are not pregnant. If in doubt, have a pregnancy test.

Tips on Preparing for an Operation

Elizabeth's preparations before having surgery to remove an endometrial lump in the hernia area may be helpful in your preparation.

> She says, "I couldn't find any one book on what to do before going in for an operation, so I gathered information from all over. I increased my vitamin intake—Evening Primrose oil, vitamin E and a multivitamin tablet. I took as many gentle walks and swims as I could and continued working, which I really enjoy.

"I also had more-regular acupuncture to help me cope with the pain and to boost my immune system, and I even used affirmations from Louise Hay's book (see "Further Reading" at the end of the book), writing my favorite one on a photo to take with me. I also wrote down as many questions as possible to ask the hospital staff, took the painkillers I'd been given and ate lots of good food, as well as relaxed and started taking herbal remedies a week before surgery.

"I packed the following in my bag: a new dressing gown and nightshirt, a personal stereo with a tape of relaxing music, some lavender essence, a sleeping mask, a book of short stories, plus a few other things the hospital suggested, such as a towel and moisturizer.

"Then, once I was in the hospital, I created my own environment by my bed: I put a photo on the table and a few drops of lavender essence on the pillow and had music playing quietly. One of the nurses smelled the lavender and came to chat about an aromatherapy course she'd taken. Someone else promised me she'd be there when I woke up, and the nurse who shaved me did it with so much humor and dignity that it made everything bearable. They even let me take my music softly playing all the way to the operating room, and when I woke up someone had started it playing and put it beside me.

"I can't pretend it was all smooth sailing. I didn't come out of the anesthetic very well. However, the nurses were wonderful; one held the basin for me while I vomited a little as another rubbed my back. The nurse who had done the aromatherapy also came to massage my feet and hands gently later on. I was amazed to receive such loving care. I stayed overnight and the next day went home.

"In the end, I was off work for five weeks longer than I had anticipated. This was partly due to the constipation caused by the painkillers. This is no joke, and I would recommend plenty of fruit, in particular stewed apples or cooked tomatoes, to ease this.

"One of the pages in a scrapbook I made also contained a list of things to look forward to—such as a friend's wedding, my brother's baby arriving and a class in pottery. Certainly, focusing on this helped me to plan ahead, as well as accept my daily progress. My colleagues sent me a large container of plants, which made me take a daily walk to and from the kitchen to water them!

"I also had stashed a few meals in the freezer and filled up the pantry with foods and juices I love, and my family was very helpful with the shopping, changing sheets as well as giving lots of love. The key is to be *organized!*"

What to Ask after the Operation

When you have recovered from your operation, it is important to ask the surgeon exactly what has been done. This is often done at a follow-up appointment, if not at the time you are in the hospital. But even then, women are often given insufficient information about their problem. You might want to avoid this by at least asking the following questions:

- What degree of endometriosis was found?
- Were there any adhesions?
- Were the bowel, bladder or reproductive organs affected in any way?
- Is any further treatment needed?
- What are the advantages and disadvantages of this treatment?

It might be well worthwhile making a list (perhaps even keeping a notebook about your surgery and the aftermath), so that you don't forget!

CHAPTER TEN

Hysterectomy

General Information

What Is a Hysterectomy?

A *hysterectomy* is the surgical removal of the uterus (womb). It is done either through an incision in the abdominal wall or vaginally. About 19.5 percent of adult women in the United States have had a hysterectomy.

Why Have a Hysterectomy?

A hysterectomy is usually only advised for older women who have already completed their childbearing. However, some young women with severe endometriosis opt to have one when all other treatments have failed. It is usually advised in the following circumstances:

- If your uterus is getting bigger, causing you circulatory problems or difficulties going to the bathroom

- If you have severe pelvic pain
- If you haven't responded to other treatments
- If the quality of your life is severely affected by uterine problems

What Are the Advantages of Having a Hysterectomy?

- It can greatly relieve endometriosis pain.
- You no longer have to put up with PMS and heavy periods.
- You never again need to have pap smears.
- It may increase your sex drive because you are no longer plagued by pain—some women even say their orgasms improve!
- You no longer need to use contraceptives.

What Are the Disadvantages?

- It isn't reversible.
- It can affect your sex life adversely—some women complain of less sensation during orgasm.
- If your ovaries are removed, you immediately become menopausal, which can lead to depression, lowered sex drive and problems associated with menopause (such as vaginal dryness).
- Even when the ovaries remain, some women may experience menopause slightly earlier following a hysterectomy.
- You may suffer emotionally because of loss of your childbearing ability.

Irene, who had had a hysterectomy at 38, two years later recalls, "Afterward I found myself looking wistfully at little children and went through a sort of mourning for the loss of my ability to conceive. It took me a while to realize that I was at an age when I would probably not choose to have a child, in any case, for health reasons—but the hysterectomy still preyed on my mind, now and then."

What Should You Bear in Mind When Deciding?

It is a good idea to have counseling both before and after a hysterectomy. Studies show that women who make the decision after sufficient counseling tend to suffer fewer emotional problems afterward. If you are nearing menopause, you might decide you would prefer to wait for it to occur naturally. You should contact your physician, HMO or community women's health clinic for information on counseling.

What Happens During a Hysterectomy?

There are several types of hysterectomy. Included here are brief descriptions:

A Total Abdominal Hysterectomy (TAH)

The removal of your uterus and cervix is called a total abdominal hysterectomy. It usually involves having a horizontal, bikini-line incision. However, when there are other complications (such as an ovarian cyst or a previous vertical scar from a Cesarean delivery), a vertical scar may be needed instead. You are also given a catheter, a flexible tube that is inserted into the bladder during the operation to drain your bladder; this may stay in place for a few days afterward so that you don't have to worry about going to the bathroom (some women say this can feel quite uncomfortable).

The surgeon then carefully cuts the uterus away from its ligaments and blood vessels, and seals them up by clamping them off. If you are keeping your ovaries, the fallopian tubes will also be separated from the uterus and clamped off. The cervix is then cut away from the vagina, which frees the uterus, allowing it to be lifted out and sent for examination. The hole where the cervix was is then stitched up. If the ovaries are left intact (sometimes one is removed), they may be stitched to the pelvic wall to avoid the possibility of their getting in the way during intercourse. Sometimes a drain is left in for a few days to get rid of any remaining debris or blood. The usual hospital stay is about one week, or longer if complications arise.

"I Had a Hysterectomy"

Christine, who is 36 with two children, says, "I went in the day before the hysterectomy and had all the usual checks done. After midnight I wasn't allowed anything to eat or drink. In the morning I was given a premedication and was taken to the operating room. I think it took about an hour and a half, and when I woke up I cried with relief. I felt peaceful and restful, and no longer all twisted up inside. I couldn't stop thanking the medical staff!

"I had a special drip going into my arm, with a button I could press to give myself painkillers, and I had an oxygen mask nearby because I was a little faint. After that, I slept most of the day. Fortunately, I was able to pass urine, though they give you a catheter if you have difficulty. I was also dosed with a mild laxative, to help me have an easier bowel movement. They taught me to cough with a rolled-up towel in front of my abdomen so that I wouldn't strain the scar.

"The wound site had a drain on it and the stitches were very well done. I found my appetite gradually returned, but for the first six weeks I couldn't do much. Friends from my local church helped me out at home, and my sister took the kids for several weeks. But it took me a good six months before I felt calmed down and stable.

"I'm really glad I had the hysterectomy, because I've put on weight since (I was too thin before), and now I only get twinges of pain (whereas before I was in pain all the time). I used to have to fight just to make my children's sandwiches. I remember my small daughter seeing me in bed all day saying, 'Poor Mommy, in bed all the time.' Now she's got the chance to have a real mom who can even do the vacuuming and braid her hair before school!"

A Subtotal or Partial Hysterectomy

This surgery entails removing the uterus while leaving the cervix in place. The advantage of this is procedure is that it is an easier operation to perform and there is less risk of complications afterward. It may also be performed if the cervix is too difficult to remove owing to adhesions. However, women who have had this operation still need to have cervical pap smears, because they remain at risk for cervical cancer.

Wertheim's Hysterectomy

Usually this surgery is only performed in cancer cases, but it is occasionally used to treat advanced endometriosis. It involves a more widespread removal of organs and tissue—not just the uterus and cervix, but also the uterine broad ligament, the ovaries and the fallopian tubes, plus any lymph glands and fatty tissues that are at risk.

> Rosa, 48, underwent a Wertheim's hysterectomy when she was 40 after the discovery of endometriosis that was partially blocking her bowel and because of multiple small cysts on the ovary. She says: "When I had the hysterectomy I couldn't understand why the other women in the hospital were recovering more quickly than I was. Then the surgeon explained that the endometriosis had been so bad that he'd had to take out everything he possibly could, including the ligaments holding the uterus in place, and that the whole operation had involved more than 200 internal stitches. It was no *wonder* I felt so ill!"

Vaginal Hysterectomy

A vaginal hysterectomy means that the whole operation is performed through the vagina, thus leaving no abdominal scar. It should also mean a shorter stay in hospital (of three to five days, as opposed to four to seven days for a TAH) and a quicker recovery time (five weeks, as opposed to six to eight weeks for a TAH). The vagina may also be tightened during the operation, and the bladder treated for stress incontinence. However, this operation isn't suitable for women who have dense adhesions.

The Laparoscopically Assisted Hysterectomy

This is a vaginal hysterectomy carried out using a laparoscope. With this technique, three small cuts are made in the abdomen through which the viewing device and the surgeon's instruments are passed. The stomach is also pumped with gas to help the surgeon see the organs more clearly. During the operation the surgeon may also divide any adhesions, as well as cut away the uterus and ovaries (if necessary). The gas is then expelled, and the uterus and ovaries are removed through the vagina.

Should I Have My Ovaries Removed?

Removal of the ovaries is known as an *oophorectomy* if one ovary is removed, or a *bilateral oophorectomy* if both are removed. The operation causes the immediate onset of menopause. Nevertheless, a lot of endometriosis sufferers choose to have their ovaries removed, because this is more likely to rid them of their pain by stopping the monthly cycle. The reason for this is that the ovaries produce estrogen, one of the main female hormones that stimulates the patches of endometriosis.

If your uterus is removed, you no longer have menstrual periods. However, if your ovaries are kept, any remaining patches of endometriosis can *still* be stimulated every month, causing pain and sometimes creating the same period-like symptoms you experienced before (such as PMS, stomach cramps and so on). Women who have had a hysterectomy but whose ovaries have remained have a 13 percent chance that endometriosis will recur within three years.

Many women say that losing their ovaries is even more traumatic than losing their uterus.

> Sally recalls: "I wasn't as upset about losing my uterus because I had two children and I'd already been sterilized, but I *was* upset about losing my ovaries. I felt as though I had lost my femininity and went through a phase of putting very heavy makeup and wearing extra-frilly dresses to try to compensate for it. Fortunately, this feeling began to fade over time and I eventually adjusted."

After the Operation

A hysterectomy is a relatively safe operation with a death rate of about one out of every 1,000. But studies show that complications occur in between 25 and 50 percent of the cases. These are mostly minor problems (such as urinary tract infections, urinary retention, pelvic abscesses, or pain during intercourse). The more serious complications include hemorrhages, damage to other organs and blood clots (although these are very rare!).

Recovery Time

Doctors advise you not to lift things for at least six weeks after the operation, and they say that it will take up to eight weeks to recover.

Every woman is different, so don't worry if you need longer for your recovery time. You also ought to allow time for the emotional adjustment: many women report it taking up to a year to get used to living without a uterus.

When Can I Have Sex Again?

Most women worry about when they will be able to resume their sex life. Again this varies, although doctors say it's as soon as the discharge and swelling have settled down, or after your first six week checkup. The simple rules are:

- Don't hurry—take your time.
- Stop if anything hurts.
- Experiment with different positions to find out which is comfortable.
- Use gels such as KY jelly and pessaries if you have lubrication problems.
- Pelvic exercises and live fresh yogurt (unflavored and sugarless, of course!) applied to the vagina are also supposed to help (see Chapter 6 for pelvic exercises).

Hysterectomy and Menopause

Menopause, often referred to as "the change of life," is the time when your last period occurs. This is seldom clear-cut: periods can come and go for a few years after the first irregularity in your cycle. Menopause is the result of the ovaries running out of eggs. For most women, this happens between the ages of 45 and 55. If you've had a hysterectomy and your ovaries have been left in place, you may be one of the 25 percent who experience menopausal symptoms within two years of having the operation. But when both ovaries are removed during surgery, menopause usually occurs very rapidly.

What Are the Symptoms?

Most of the symptoms are related to the withdrawal of estrogen and the effect of increasing levels of the FSH (see Chapter 1) that result. The most common symptom is *hot flashes,* experienced by nearly 80 percent of menopausal women. Other immediate effects might include *night sweats* and *frequent urination.*

More long-term effects include: dryness of the vagina and of the skin in general, a loss of sex drive, and problems with intercourse due to the thinning of vaginal walls, making them sore and susceptible to tearing.

Hysterectomy and Hormone Replacement Therapy (HRT)

What Is HRT Treatment?

Hormone replacement therapy (HRT) involves taking, in synthetic form, some of the hormones that your ovaries have stopped making (normally, estrogen and progesterone).

Why Take HRT?

- It can relieve some of the symptoms of menopause.

- It helps prevent osteoporosis, a thinning of the bones caused by the demineralization (primarily calcium) of bone, often attributed to a lack of estrogen.

Self-Help for Hot Flashes

- Wear layers of light clothing that can be easily removed as you get warmer and replaced as you cool down.

- Avoid synthetic materials, because they prevent the air from circulating freely.

- Cut down on caffeine drinks, alcohol, spicy food and smoking—all of which are thought to trigger hot flashes.

- Try frequent and brief lukewarm showers rather than a bath.

- Exercise regularly.

- Take vitamin E (200–400 IU each day), which may help excessive hot flashes and sweats.

- Try any of the capsules now on the market containing trace elements and vitamins especially for menopause.

- For night sweats, place a cotton towel over your lower bed sheet to absorb extra perspiration.

- Research has shown that it offers some protection against heart attacks and strokes.

What Are the Risks of HRT?

Some women have been on hormone replacement therapy for over 20 years, and evidence shows that it is safe for most users. However, it is still important to tell your doctor that you have endometriosis (this will affect the choice of drugs prescribed) or if any of the following problems apply to you:

- You or any of your close family has had breast cancer.

- You have had cancer of the uterus or ovaries.

- You've had large fibroids.

- You have active endometriosis.

- You have a history of thrombosis or blood clots.

- You are a heavy smoker.

Or if you suffer from any of the following:

- Severe migraine headaches

- High blood pressure

- Diabetes

- Liver disease

- Gallstones

- Malignant melanoma

- Otosclerosis (an ear condition that progressively causes deafness)

- Multiple sclerosis

- Porphyria (a hereditary disease)

What Are the Disadvantages of HRT?

Many women report unpleasant side effects, although some experience only a few, or find that they disappear after a while. Some side effects may be eliminated by changing to a different brand, type or dosage of HRT.

The common side effects are:

- Breast soreness

- Weight gain

- Headaches

- Bloating

- Muscle cramps

- Nausea

- Fluid retention
- Swollen ankles
- Increased blood pressure
- Dizziness
- Depression

Which HRT Should I Take?

HRT comes in several forms. It can be swallowed as tablets, applied to the skin in a patch form or as a gel, placed under the skin in implants or inserted into the vagina as a cream or pessary.

Many types of hormone replacement therapies are available. It is a good idea to discuss with your physician which symptoms are bothering you, since some treatments are better than others for particular problems.

Take note! Some women who haven't yet reached menopause are being prescribed low-dose hormone replacement therapy as a way of counteracting some of the effects of drug treatment (see Chapter 8).

Endometriosis After a Hysterectomy

Once the ovaries have been removed, you would expect your problems with endometriosis to be over. However, some women do still have difficulties. It is thought that small amounts of the ovary are sometimes left behind and continue to produce estrogen. Also, the adrenal glands may still produce sex hormones that can be converted into estrogen by fatty tissue.

> Lisa, a 57-year-old retired civil servant, says: "When I was recovering from my hysterectomy I was dismayed to find that, besides the pain of the operation, the original pain was still there. I was immediately given HRT patches, but this just made me feel worse. I got terrible headaches. Eventually I got into such a state that I forgot to change the patches, which actually made the headaches go away and reduced the pain. I told my

doctor and eventually she tailor-made a hormone replacement patch for me that included progesterone, which she said would counteract the effects of the estrogen. I finally got relief."

Livial—The New Hormone Replacement Therapy

Livial (or *Tibolone*) is the first single substance to combine the actions of the three sex hormones estrogen, progesterone and testosterone. It is not usually prescribed until a year after the last period, to give the uterine lining time to break down. It doesn't stimulate the endometrium, and so regular monthly bleeding on this form of HRT is avoided. It is supposed to be good for several reasons: it improves vaginal and urinary skin quality, which makes intercourse less painful; it reduces the loss of bone density; and it has no adverse effects on cholesterol or blood-clotting factors. It is thought to be a good drug to use following a hysterectomy. Unfortunately, it is not presently available in the United States, but is available in Great Britain.

The Natural Progesterone Debate

One school of thought now suggests that it is extra progesterone, not estrogen, that needs to be given during menopause since, at this time, progesterone production drops to almost nothing, whereas small amounts of estrogen are still made. Most HRT formulas do include synthetic progesterone, but researchers such as Dr. John Lee believe that it is very different from the natural hormone progesterone. He recommends natural progesterone cream to many of his patients because he believes it can actually restore bone growth. Some of his patients have reported that their PMS and water retention vanished while using the progesterone cream.

Many fresh foods contain progesterone-like ingredients. Mexican yam, for instance, contains diosgenin, a substance that needs only one change to become progesterone itself. However, how Mexican yam works on the body is not yet known. You can obtain wild yam progesterone as a cream, oil, tablet or capsule over the counter at some health food stores or through herbalists.

CHAPTER ELEVEN

A Better Understanding?

Is There a Cure?

At the moment there is no cure for endometriosis. As you have learned over the course of this book, most of the treatments focus on getting rid of the pain, restoring fertility and managing the illness. On the positive side, endometriosis does not necessarily get worse over time. If that were so, many older women would be suffering from severe endometriosis. In fact, research suggests that endometriosis naturally resolves itself in 25 percent of cases, and that in 50 percent of cases it gradually moves from an active to a more passive, tolerable form.

How Often Does It Return?

Unfortunately, none of the treatments is foolproof. Hormonal treatments successfully treat pain in 85 percent of cases, but this is not a permanent cure. Only 50 percent of women with endometriosis are helped by hormonal treatment, because the cysts tend to grow back once treatment ends. The exact recurrence rate of endometriosis after conservative surgery is not known (rates vary, because of the lack of specific long-term studies). Recurrence rates after a hysterectomy if the ovaries remain is 13 percent within three years and 40 percent after five years; in a few cases, endometriosis returns even after the ovaries have been removed.

What You Do If It Returns

If endometriosis returns, you may need to undergo a second treatment. But usually the recurrence must first be diagnosed to make certain the pain is not caused by post surgical adhesions, pelvic inflammation or adenomyosis (hot spots in the uterine wall; see Chapter 1). As with the first treatment, your symptoms, the extent of the disease, your desire to have children, as well as other complications, all need to be taken into consideration when deciding what course to follow.

Learning to Live with It

Emotionally, a recurrence can be very difficult to handle. We often hang on to the belief that everything will be okay once we have had a treatment. We may put total trust in the medical establishment, or in a combination of surgical or drug intervention and complementary, holistic therapies. Despite all our efforts, we may feel we have failed in some way if endometriosis returns. On top of that, we may have to deal with the feelings of others.

> Jackie says: "One difficulty can be the expectation of others. Friends, relatives and colleagues are expecting the treatment to *work,* and initially they don't expect the endometriosis to return—so it becomes a process of an all-around education both of yourself and of people you're close to."

It can be extremely difficult to come to terms with the fact that you have a disease that may limit you in various ways—ways that could get better or worse with time. You need to remind yourself that endometriosis isn't the *whole* of you, and that you can't just wait for a mythical future date when everything will be fine. You have to get on with your life and make decisions in the here-and-now.

> Everyone has different ways of doing this. Jackie has a little useful advice on this subject: "One thing I have learned is persistence, and to glean all the information I can. As my community's endo society slogan goes, 'Never give up'—and I won't.
>
> "Sometimes I visualize to myself a little cartoon entitled 'Pain relief: Shoot your doctor!' It just helps during the frustrating times. I'm not an aggressive person—just more assertive!"

And if all else fails, remember that you are in good company. The following people have all managed to cope with endometriosis and lead fulfilling lives (and there are many more of us out there!): actress Marilyn Monroe, tennis player Mary Jo Fernandez and writer Hilary Mantels.

Your Action Plan

1. Don't accept that painful periods are normal.

2. Don't be embarrassed to discuss the symptoms.

3. Ask for explanations—again and again.

4. Keep a diary of events, detailing your pain, your periods and any associated problems.

5. If all else fails, consider changing your doctor or specialist.

6. Inform yourself. Gather as much information as you can from doctors and nurses, from other sufferers and from self-help groups.

Remember there is light at the end of the tunnel. And finally, good luck!

Further Reading

Ballweg, Mary Lou (editor), Endometriosis Association, *The Endometriosis Sourcebook: The Definitive Guide to Current Treatment Options, the Latest Research, Common Myths About the Disease and Coping Strategies*. Hill and Wang, 1995.

Brown, Ellen Hodgson, *Breezing Through the Change: Managing Menopause Naturally*. North Atlantic Books, 1994.

Chaitow, Leon, *Candida Albicans: Could Yeast be Your Problem?* Thorsons, 1995.

Haas, Adelaide, Susan L. Puretz, *The Woman's Guide to Hysterectomy: Expectations & Options*. Celestial Arts, 1995.

Hall, Doriel, *Discover Meditation*. Ulysses Press, 1997.

Hay, Louise, *You Can Heal Your Life*. Hay House, 1994.

Lark, Susan M., *Dr. Susan Lark's the Estrogen Decision Self Help Book: A Complete Guide for Relief of Menopausal Symptoms Through Hormonal Replacement and Alternatives*. Celestial Arts, 1996.

Levine, Stephen, *Guided Meditations, Explorations and Healing*. Double Day, 1991.

Naylor, Nicola, *Discover Essential Oils*. Ulysses Press, 1998.

Oxenford, Rosalind, *Discover Reflexology*. Ulysses Press, 1997.

Sadler, Jan, *Natural Pain Relief — A Practical Handbook of Self-Help*. Element Books, 1997.

Siegel, Bernie, *Love, Medicine and Miracles*. HarperCollins, 1990.

Sneddon, Pete, and Paolo Coseschi, *Discover Osteopathy*. Ulysses Press, 1997.

Storch, M., *How to Relieve Cramps and Other Menstrual Problems*. Workman, 1982.

Sutton, Catherine, *Discover Shiatsu*. Ulysses Press, 1998

Trickett, Shirley, *Anxiety & Depression*. Ulysses Press, 1997.

Trickett, Shirley, *Free Yourself from Tranquilizers & Sleeping Pills*. Ulysses Press, 1997.

Winston, Robert, *Getting Pregnant*. Pan, 1993.

The New Our Bodies, Ourselves: A Book by and for Women. The Boston Women's Health Book Collective, 1996.

Useful Addresses

Endometriosis Organizations

Endometriosis Association Education Support Research
International Headquarters
8585 North 76th Place
Milwaukee, WI 53223
phone: 414-355-2200
fax: 414-355-6065
web site: http://www.endometriosisassn.org

American Society for Reproductive Medicine
Washington Office
409 12th Street, SW, Suite 203
Washington, DC 20024-2152
phone: 205-978-5000
fax: 205-978-5005
e-mail: asrm@asrm.com
web site: http://www.asrm.com

Complementary Medicine

National Institutes of Health–
Office of Alternative Medicine Clearinghouse
P.O. Box 8218
Silver Springs, Maryland 20907-8218
phone: 888-644-6226
TTY/TDY: 888-644-6226
fax: 301-495-4957

American Holistic Health Association
P.O. Box 17400
Anaheim, CA 92817
phone: 714-779-6152
e-mail: ahha@healthy.net
web page: http://ahha.org

American Holistic Medical Association
6728 Old McLean Village Drive
McLean, VA 22101
phone: 703-556-9728
fax: 703-556-8729
web page: http://www.ahmaholistic.com

Osteopathy Resources

American Osteopathic Association (AOA)
142 East Ontario Street
Chicago, IL 60611-2864
phone: 312-280-5800

American Academy of Osteopathy (AAO)
3500 DePauw Boulevard, Suite 1080
Indianapolis, IN 46268-1136
phone: 317-879-1881

Coping Strategies

Pain Management Centers

The American Chronic Pain Association
P.O. Box 859
Rocklin, CA 95677
phone: 916-632-0922

The American Pain Society
4700 West Lake Avenue
Glenview, IL 60025
phone: 847-375-4715
fax: 847-375-4777
e-mail: info@ampainsoc.org
web site: http://www.ampainsoc.org

Smoking

American Cancer Society
phone: 800-227-2345
web site: http://www.cancer.org

American Lung Association
1740 Broadway
New York, NY 10019
phone: 800-586-4872
web site: http://www.lungusa.org

Eating Disorders

National Eating Disorders Association
6655 South Yale Avenue
Tulsa, OK 74136
phone: 918-481-4044

Index

Ulysses Press Health Books

A Natural Approach Books

Written in a friendly, nontechnical style, *A Natural Approach* books address specific health issues and show you how to take an active part in your own treatment. Whether you suffer from panic attacks, endometriosis or depression, each book will provide you with a thorough understanding of your condition and detail organic solutions that offer immediate relief for your symptoms and effectively remedy their underlying causes.

Believing that disease is more than a combination of symptoms, these books offer integrated mind/body programs that take a positive, preventative approach. Since traditional drug therapy is not always the best solution (and can sometimes be the problem), these guides show how to use alternative treatments to supplement or replace conventional medicine.

ANXIETY & DEPRESSION
ISBN 1-56975-118-8, 144 pp, $9.95

ENDOMETRIOSIS
ISBN 1-56975-088-2, 184 pp, $9.95

FREE YOURSELF FROM TRANQUILIZERS
& SLEEPING PILLS
ISBN 1-56975-074-2, 192 pp, $9.95

IRRITABLE BLADDER & INCONTINENCE
ISBN 1-56975-089-0, 108 pp, $8.95

IRRITABLE BOWEL SYNDROME
ISBN 1-56975-030-0, 240 pp, $11.95

MIGRAINES
ISBN 1-56975-140-4, 156 pp, $8.95

PANIC ATTACKS
ISBN 1-56975-045-9, 148 pp, $8.95

The Natural Healer Books

As home remedies and alternative treatments become increasingly accepted into the medical mainstream, people want information—not just hype and unproven claims—about the remedies they see in health food stores. *The Natural Healer* books detail how these natural remedies have been used throughout history and how to safely incorporate them into an overall plan for maintaining good health.

CIDER VINEGAR
ISBN 1-56975-141-2, 120 pp, $8.95

GARLIC
ISBN 1-56975-097-1, 120 pp, $8.95

Discover Handbooks

Easy to follow and authoritative, *Discover Handbooks* reveal an array of alternative therapies from around the world and demonstrate how to incorporate them into a program of good health.

Each book opens with information on the history and principles of the particular technique, then presents practical and straightforward guidance on ways in which it can be applied. Offering the tools needed to achieve and maintain an optimal state of health, the approach is one of personal improvement and self-reliance. Each of the books features: an introduction to the discipline; an explanation of its philosophy; step-by-step guide to its implementation; clear diagrams and charts; and case studies.

DISCOVER AYURVEDA
ISBN 1-56975-081-5, 128 pp, $8.95

DISCOVER COLOR THERAPY
ISBN 1-56975-093-9, 144 pp, $8.95

DISCOVER ESSENTIAL OILS
ISBN 1-56975-080-7, 128 pp, $8.95

DISCOVER FLOWER ESSENCES
ISBN 1-56975-099-8, 120 pp, $8.95

DISCOVER MEDITATION
ISBN 1-56975-113-7, 144 pp, $8.95

DISCOVER NUTRITIONAL THERAPY
ISBN 1-56975-135-8, 120 pp, $8.95

DISCOVER OSTEOPATHY
ISBN 1-56975-115-3, 132 pp, $8.95

DISCOVER REFLEXOLOGY
ISBN 1-56975-112-9, 132 pp, $8.95

DISCOVER SHIATSU
ISBN 1-56975-082-3, 128 pp, $8.95

The Ancient and Healing Arts Books

The Ancient and Healing Arts books recount the development of healing art forms that have been used for thousands of years. Beautifully illustrated with full color on every page, they discuss the benefits of these time-honored techniques and offer detailed instructions on their use.

THE ANCIENT AND HEALING ART OF
AROMATHERAPY
ISBN 1-56975-094-7, 96 pp, $14.95

THE ANCIENT AND HEALING ART OF
CHINESE HERBALISM
ISBN 1-56975-139-0, 96 pp, $14.95

Other Health Titles

THE BOOK OF KOMBUCHA
ISBN 1-56975-049-1, 160 pp, $11.95
Explains the benefits of and addresses concerns about Kombucha, the widely used Chinese "tea mushroom."

HEPATITIS C: A PERSONAL GUIDE TO GOOD HEALTH
ISBN 1-56975-091-2, 172 pp, $12.95
Identifies the causes and symptoms of hepatitis C and presents conventional and alternative treatments for coping with the disease.

KNOW YOUR BODY: THE ATLAS OF ANATOMY
ISBN 1-56975-021-1, 160 pp, $12.95
Presents a full-color guide to the structure of the human body.

MOOD FOODS
ISBN 1-56975-023-8, 192 pp, $9.95
Shows how the foods you eat influence your emotions and behavior.

YOUR NATURAL PREGNANCY: A GUIDE TO COMPLEMENTARY THERAPIES
ISBN 1-56975-059-9, 240 pp, $16.95
Details alternative therapies ranging from aromatherapy to yoga that can benefit pregnant women.

———————

To order these books call 800-377-2542, fax 510-601-8307 or write to Ulysses Press, P.O. Box 3440, Berkeley, CA 94703-3440. All retail orders are shipped free of charge. California residents must include sales tax. Allow two to three weeks for delivery.

About the Author

JO MEARS graduated from University College, London, in 1984 and then trained as a journalist at the London College of Printing. She worked for The Press Association, *The Daily Mirror* and *Me* magazine before becoming a freelance writer. She now regularly contributes health articles to British newspapers and magazines such as *Woman's Own* and *New Woman*.